Surviving Exercise

Judy Alter

Surviving Exercise

Judy Alter's
Safe and Sane
Exercise Program

Illustrations by
Rochelle Robkin

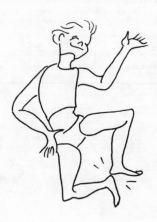

Houghton Mifflin Company · Boston

For information about permission to reproduce selections
from this book, write to Permissions, Houghton Mifflin
Company, 2 Park Street, Boston, Massachusetts 02108.

Library of Congress Cataloging in Publication Data
Alter, Judy.
   Surviving exercise.
      1. Exercise.   2. Exercise—Safety measures.
I. Robkin, Rochelle.   II. Title.
RA781.A564 1983   613.7'1   82-21319
ISBN 0-395-33112-9
ISBN 0-395-50073-7 (pbk.)

Printed in the United States of America

S 18 17 16 15 14 13 12 11 10

Contents

Foreword vii
Preface ix

1. How to Work Out Without Killing Yourself 1
   Safe Exercise

2. The Basic Don'ts for Readiness Exercises 14

3. Your Neck 27

4. Your Arms and Shoulders 35

5. Your Back, Waist, and Stomach Area 46

6. Your Legs 58
   Your Calf
   The Back of Your Thigh
   Stretching the Front of Your Thigh
   Strengthening the Front of Your Thigh
   Stretching the Upper Hip
   Your Inner Thigh

7. Your Feet 88

8.   Common Running and Walking
     Mistakes 91
         Safe Running and Walking: A Checklist

9.   In Case of Injury 98

10. Summary 100
         Readiness Exercises for Your Legs
         Readiness Exercises for Your Upper Body
         Readiness Exercises for General Well-Being
         The Don'ts and Do's of Exercise

     Acknowledgments 111

     Recommended Books for
     Injury Prevention 113

Foreword

It was indeed a pleasure to review this book, *Surviving Exercise*. Ms. Alter has distilled years of exposure to good — and bad — exercise from her own experiences as a dancer, teacher, and exercise leader; and she has produced a clear, concise, and well-illustrated guide to the do's and don'ts of floor exercise.

She quite properly decries the paradox that the pursuit of better health through exercise too often results in unnecessary injury — and impaired health. She additionally notes the need for preventive medicine and preventive exercise in the fields of fitness and sports medicine.

Many exercise books are now available that present a variety of pushes, pulls, twists, and rolls to the reader, often without evident physiological basis and often inadequately explained. Too often, the author will emphasize either stretching or strengthening exercises, to the exclusion of one or the other aspect of musculoskeletal conditioning. There is also a growing romance with machines and "exercise systems" in the fitness and exercise field, with, all too often, inadequate thought given to the objectives of these exercises.

Ms. Alter emphasizes both that proper conditioning is a combination of both strengthening and stretching and that concentrating on one to the exclusion of the other is to invite injury. She also notes that exercises in sports such as biking, swimming, or running can cause imbalances in the muscles and joints of the body that require additional supplemental exercises in order to prevent injury.

In addition to emphasizing proper exercise, the author repeatedly emphasizes the mistakes that can be made in an exercise program. This is a particularly advantageous aspect of this book, further reflecting the wealth of experience that the author has had in exercise instruction.

I have found this little gem of a book useful in dealing with my athletes and dancers, who often know what they wish their body to do but do not necessarily know how to achieve it. This book can be recommended as an exercise guide by the physician, physical therapist, or exercise leader, to patients or clients who need a safe and clear introduction to exercise.

Lyle J. Micheli, M.D.

Director, Division of Sports Medicine at
Children's Hospital Medical Center, Boston, and
Vice President for Medicine,
American College of Sports Medicine

Preface

No! Pain is not necessary for exercise gain. This book screams: Stop if it hurts! Pain is a life-saving signal to you to stop the exercise or activity you are doing. You probably already know that and instinctively have stopped doing exercises that hurt you or made you uncomfortable. Actually, you could write a major part of this book because you know which exercises you don't like to do. Yet you don't want to be an exercise dropout. You don't have to quit your aerobic workouts or shaping-up regimes. You can substitute safe "readying" exercises for the harmful ones, or correct them and enjoy greater safety in your life-enhancing exercise times.

Surviving Exercise tells you why some of the popular exercises are harmful or useless. But instead of only saying, "No! Stop the painful ones!" it provides you with exercises that *really* work either to stretch your muscles properly or strengthen your muscles efficiently. Most important, this book tells you how to protect your body/yourself from injury during the times when you get ready to run or play a game, and during your activity.

All that in one little book? Yes. Here are safe and sane exercises for your neck, shoulders, abdominal muscles, for your hips, thighs, calves, and feet. Here are guidelines for safe walking and running, for weightlifting, for bending over. And here are three exercise programs — short (5 minutes), medium (9 minutes), and longer (20 minutes) — that you can use before and after all physical activity.

Surviving Exercise offers you a balance of outside information from experts and inside information from your own body. This information can enable you to go beyond this book and learn to judge for yourself what is best for your muscles. The guidelines presented in *Surviving Exercise* give you a means of correcting any exercise you know. You can, once and for all, trust the signals your muscles are sending you when you hold a position in order to stretch a specific muscle group, or move slowly up and down against gravity to gain strength in that muscle group. You will understand why you should feel release of tension while stretching, feel warm fatigue while strengthening, and **always stop if it hurts!**

There are ways of knowing what works for your body and what does not. For years, teachers of anatomy, physical education, physical therapy, and kinesiology have been saying, "Stop if it hurts!" "Don't bounce, don't back arch, don't lock your knees!" For years, the harm of double leg lifts, deep knee bends, fast sit-ups, and prone arches has been known. But the old harmful practices persist in exercise programs, and people continue to hurt themselves doing the old traditional exercises.

Years ago, as a dance student, I did all the techniques my dance teachers told me to do, even if my body hurt from doing them. I sustained a number of serious and not-so-serious injuries, but like most people who get used to physical exercise of any sort, I would not stop dancing or dance training, even if it hurt me. Once I began to teach dance, my goal became to prevent pain and injury. I had learned from my courses in anatomy and kinesiology (the study of human movement) that it should be possible to exercise without becoming sore, and I found, through practice, that this is true.

Another source from which I learned to prevent injury was my students' questions, revealing the specific needs of each unique body. The open atmosphere in my classes helped bring about a number of exciting discoveries, some of which are in this book. The most important discovery was that my students and I could dance without painful injuries, and everyone experienced progress. The "tight" students became more flexible and the flexible students gained more strength. All of them grew better coordinated and their movements more fluid. And very few students sustained any injuries.

After a few years of teaching dance, I began to get requests from the parents of my students to help them work out muscle cramps, or get relief from back pain, or build up enough strength to run. This experience enabled me to apply my dance injury-prevention techniques to nondancers. I learned as much from my nondance clients as I learned from my dance students. This book is the result of that combined experience.

Also I learned about these injury-prevention techniques from reading medical literature. I had access to the medical libraries of Tufts University, Boston University, Harvard University, and the University of Wisconsin—Madison. With the use of MEDLINE, the computer data bank of medical literature, I was able to search specifically for articles about injuries of the knee, ankle, back, and neck. I found that dance and sport injuries had similar causes and, of course, similarly devastating results when careers were interrupted or ended prematurely. Most of the medical literature focused on treatment of injuries and rehabilitation after recovery, but very little of it focused on prevention or even possible specific causes other than impact.

Everyone is interested in injury prevention. I give 35–40 workshops across the country each year to groups of lay people, dance teachers, professional dancers, coaches, runners, doctors and physical therapists, and physical education teachers from elementary schools, junior and senior high schools, and colleges. Regional and national sports and dance organizations have invited me back to review and deepen their understanding of the exercises and information I have taught them previously. *Surviving Exercise* contains the material that I present in these workshops. After the workshops and in letters I receive, people tell me stories of their recovery from pain and injury. They describe their improved performance, and they celebrate their return to full activity because of this information. There is a very large community of people who are glad to give up harmful, ouch!-producing exercises and replace them with ones that produce actual results they want — usefully strong muscles that have the range of motion they are intended to have.

Here are some stories about the value of these exercises. An automobile mechanic had such pain in his neck that he became unable to repair cars. I had him do the three shoulder stretches and neck stretches and strengthening exercises in this book. They eliminated his pain during the session, and he now starts and ends his working day with these exercises and is able to continue earning his living.

I received a letter from a professional golfer in Florida, telling me that he had stopped having severe back and knee pain after using the "door frame pull" and the correct hamstring stretches, which he learned from this book. Another message came from Switzerland. An American mountain climber sent a postcard thanking me for my stretching exercises. They enabled him to keep his muscles responsive to the challenges of climbing.

The shoulder and neck stretches have helped two concert pianists, a violinist, and a wrestler to recover from severe pain and resume their activities on the day I gave them the exercises to do. The back pain suffered by a librarian and a secretary was markedly lessened after almost two years of intense discomfort.

Here is another success story, about a college student who is a member of the women's soccer team at the University of Wisconsin–Madison. She had broken her ankle in the spring, had been in a cast for ten weeks, and came to see me in the summer. She said her coach didn't expect her to play for a year, but she missed playing so much that she wanted to train and maybe speed up the recovery period. She also had very loose ligaments so she had never felt the need to stretch her muscles. She walked and ran with her feet pointing out, and so her ankle was weakened by her daily habits. I taught her both stretching and strengthening exercises for her legs, ankles, and toes. I had her begin to jump rope in front of a mirror to monitor the alignment of her feet, ankles, and knees. By the middle of the fall, she was able to jog without pain and soreness and began to go to soccer practices to be with the team. Her coach couldn't believe his eyes. Her form was better than ever. Her running was smoother and more efficient than he had ever seen. He even asked her to teach all her stretch and strength techniques to the entire team as part of their regular warm-up.

Using the exercises in this book, I have helped revamp high school football warm-up exercises, track-team training sessions, and aerobic dance-class preparation; and I even have an entire elementary school doing a corrected version of the Presidential Physical Fitness Program. The results that I know of are specific and individual. These exercises result in slimmer waists for men and women, better muscle tone, the elimination of back, knee, shoulder, and neck pain, and of course an enormous sense of satisfaction and feeling of well-being. I highly recommend that you try the safe ones in this book and stop doing the harmful ones. Then you will enjoy the survival benefits of healthy exercising.

Judy Alter

Los Angeles, California

P.S. My second book, *Stretch and Strengthen* (Houghton Mifflin, 1986), contains 102 safe and sane exercises and is available at bookstores. In that book there are from 3 to 8 exercises for every part of your body, graded from beginner to advanced. Because so many people have written me, asking if there are videotapes for these exercises, I am producing them. They will be sold in bookstores or you can order them by writing:

Surviving Exercise
P.O. Box 480340
Los Angeles, CA 90048-1340

1 | How to Work Out Without Killing Yourself

Yes, of course, work out! Today, it almost goes without saying: Everyone knows that exercise is important. Why? The current jogging and fitness craze stems from a clear awareness that your heart and lungs must be exercised regularly in order to be strong and to be able to handle emergencies like shock, fright, or the sudden need for speed. Regular exercise that works your heart and lungs can also help prevent heart attacks and lessen the body's susceptibility to other debilitating or fatal diseases. And, thank goodness, exercise burns calories and helps build and maintain muscle tone for all or most of your muscles. More about that on page 6, explaining balanced use of muscles. Exercise even has a therapeutic effect. People feel better after doing it because the brain secretes a tranquilizer-like substance after about ten minutes of continuous exercise. So, when regular exercisers can't get in their daily "fix," they miss it and even feel depressed. A person's entire well-being can be enhanced by regular exercise. It can be fun, challenging, and relaxing. Obviously, for all of these reasons, exercise is good for you.

But is it? What about all the injuries people get? Ankles, knees, backs, elbows, and necks get hurt. This list includes most of the body's movable joints. If exercise is so good for you, why do all these injuries occur? Because people don't know how to exercise correctly.

What is the correct way to exercise?

The safe way!

"Don't be a smart aleck," you say. "What does 'safe' mean?" The purpose of this little book is to give you a safe set of exercises for stretch and strength from head to toe, to instruct you how to do them correctly, and to explain what exercises not to do and why. This book also presents an understanding of why keeping your body moving is important for preventing and healing injury. Safe exercising is a vital means of surviving.

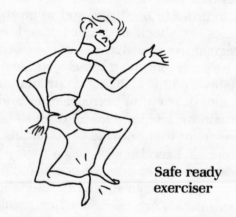

Safe ready
exerciser

Safe Exercise

The human body is built, designed, and engineered for movement. In order to stay truly fit, all the moving parts need to remain optimally mobile. What does this mean?

Body Basics

Here are some facts about the components of your body that enable you to move.

Bones

Bones support your body weight. They are rigid and are not meant to bend; nor can they move by themselves.

Joints

Joints are the places where various bones in your body meet together. Each joint has a range of movement that is determined by three factors:

1. the shapes of the bones where they meet,
2. the looseness or tightness of your ligaments, and
3. the stretchiness and strength of your muscles.

Ligaments

Ligaments hold your bones together at the joints, as a marionette's limbs are connected to its body. Though pliable, most ligaments are inelastic and only permit or re-

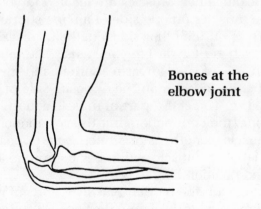

Bones at the
elbow joint

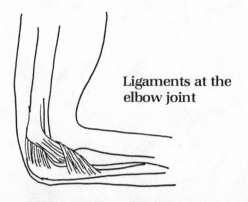

Ligaments at the elbow joint

strict movement, the way a hinge allows a door to swing open and shut. Ligaments do not contract on their own or actually move your bones.

Muscles

Your body moves by means of muscles. Muscles are elastic. On their own, muscles can only shorten and thereby pull bones together. Muscles are located in your body in sets. The muscles on one side of a bone shorten while the muscles on the other side lengthen. For example, bend your hand forward at your wrist. The muscles on the palm side of your forearm shorten, and the pull lengthens the muscles on the opposite side of your wrist and forearm. The active part of muscle action is the shortening, the contraction, but the contraction of one set of muscles lengthens or stretches an opposite set. The initiation of muscle action begins from a stretched or relaxed position.

Tendons are the harder, narrower ends of muscles and attach your muscles to your bones. Tendons look

4

very much like ligaments. They are pliable the way leather is but not elastic the way a rubber band is. You should think about them as the means by which muscles attach to bones, and not as things by themselves, as ligaments are.

So, muscles are the moving force of your body. The force of the muscle is transmitted to the bones by the tendons. Your brain thinks a movement; your nerves carry the message; the muscles move the bones. Movement almost always involves the contraction of some muscles and the stretching of others; this changes the position of the bones, which move at the joints.

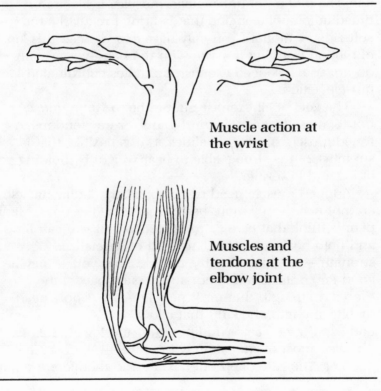

Muscle action at
the wrist

Muscles and
tendons at the
elbow joint

Safe Exercise Means a Balanced Use of Muscles

Muscles must be stretched and strengthened to be useful. Daily activity does not produce a balance of stretching and strengthening for muscles. That is why exercises are prescribed before and after most strenuous activity. Even daily walking, sitting, or bed rest unevenly stretches some muscles and tightens others.

A balance of stretch and strength is necessary to tone your muscles so that your body can move efficiently and smoothly. Muscles that are too tight or too weak cannot move your limbs in a coordinated and controlled manner. The motion of unbalanced muscles is like an untimed automobile engine that is firing irregularly; the result is jerky motion. You may have experienced this kind of motion in trying to write with the hand you usually do not use. Balanced exercise promotes coordinated muscle action.

The goal of all exercise should be to "tone" *muscles*, not to stress ligaments, grind joints, or fray tendons. A toned muscle has two qualities: 1. It is flexible, that is, stretchy. 2. It is strong, able to bear weight by holding or lifting and lowering.

A toned muscle need not be big. Large bulky muscles are not necessarily more useful than slimmer ones. Many people think that being strong means that you can lift and hold heavy weights. This kind of specialized strength — the kind that big muscles give you — may be good for contests but is not a necessary part of the everyday strength that most people need. People need mobile strength, the kind that allows you to control your body and the objects you lift, move, and lower. Bulky muscles, most often, can only hold weight in a static manner. They are often not flexible and therefore are not really toned. People with this type of muscle are called muscle-bound. Bulky muscles are not useful in activities requiring fluid or rapid motion; they can even inhibit movement.

In order for your body to thrive — to enable you to do whatever you want whenever you want — you need to provide your muscles with a balance of stretching and strengthening activities. Walking, running, biking, and swimming are all excellent activities for building and maintaining cardiovascular fitness (tone in the heart and lungs). But these activities mainly contract muscles. Over a period of time, if the contracted muscles don't get fully stretched out, the joints become vulnerable and susceptible to excess stress, which in turn leads to injury. On the other hand, some parts of your body, such as your abdominal area, mostly get stretched in daily activity. If you don't adequately strengthen this part of your body, your back and knees are more vulnerable to strain.

To prevent this series of events from occurring, here are six key instructions for surviving exercise. In preparation for any activity and following any activity:

1. Stretch muscles that you have strengthened (contracted).
2. Strengthen muscles that you have stretched.
3. **Stop** any and all activity if it hurts — "Ouch!"

Contained in the Key Instruction "**Stop** if it **Hurts**" are three more keys to Surviving Exercise:

4. Feel all muscle activity; that is, pay attention to the sensations of muscles relaxing (stretching) and contracting (strengthening), and trust your perception of these sensations.

5. Keep moving, because for muscles to be useful they must be used.

6. Be guided by the inherited and developed limits of your body.

Here now is further clarification of each of these six key instructions, starting with the last one and working back to the first.

Be guided by the inherited and developed limits of your body.

You know that you inherit your hair color, eye color, and height. Did you know that you are also programmed to develop loose or tight or average ligaments that hold your bones together? While this inherited program determines your basic ligament structure, ligaments can adapt to activity. Your structure is very important in determining how you should use your body in physical activity. Often people with loose ligaments (incorrectly called "double-jointed") think they don't need to stretch any of their muscles, and if they do try stretching, they often do not feel the stretches in their muscles. This lack of stretch sensation may result from not doing the stretches correctly, or from improper positioning of the parts of the body that are being stretched. The exercise parts of this book contain instructions on how to stretch correctly.

On the other hand, people with tight ligaments are less prone to joint injury but they often experience discomfort in their joints during exercise because unstretched muscles, when being stretched incorrectly, will cause strong stretch sensation across the joints as well as in the muscles. Both tight-ligamented and loose-ligamented people need to understand

their bodies' natural limits and to adapt their activity to
fit their bodies. This book includes guidelines for
both.

*Keep moving, because for muscles to be useful they
must be used.*
Untoned muscles are not very useful and entirely un-
used muscles atrophy. To atrophy means that they
shrink in size and lose their ability to contract with
power or relax (stretch) from their contraction. Muscles
atrophy while in a plaster cast used for immobilizing a
broken bone when it is mending. When the cast is re-
moved, these atrophied muscles, if exercised carefully and
regularly, will, in time, regain their former tone. In gen-
eral, the more regularly muscles are used, in a balanced
way, the more healthy, vital, and able to function they
will remain. The more irregularly they are used, the
greater the discomfort and pain there will be in using
them and the more vulnerable they will be to injury. Re-
cent medical practice recognizes the health-promoting
results of exercise, because doctors now instruct their
surgery patients to get up and walk as soon as possible,
within 24 hours after an operation. The recovery is faster
if a patient's entire body is kept active. This idea is true
for most injuries. Motion is healing.

*Feel all exercises in your muscles and learn to trust
your perception of strength and stretch sensations.*
When you exercise for strength or stretch you should
experience the sensations in your muscles. More than
likely, you know the feeling of stretched muscles because, like most people, you stretch after awakening from
sleep. The release of tension that stretching produces is

a strong and satisfying sensation in the muscles. *Correct stretching requires holding until the tension in the muscles releases. This usually takes about a minute,* though you may need to hold a position longer to feel the tightness of the muscle release. And you know the sensation of muscles strengthening from the fatigue of weight bearing, after, for instance, carrying a large bag of groceries up several flights of stairs. *Correct strengthening involves working muscles slowly, up and down against gravity, just a little beyond their point of fatigue.* Stretching involves active holding, and strengthening involves continuous and slow motion.

Stop any and all activity if it hurts — "Ouch!" hurts.
You know the sharp, hot stinging sensation of pain, "Ouch!" pain. A pinprick, a drop of hot oil, a hammer-hit thumb produce such strong, sudden pain. Pain is an easily recognized signal and should not be ignored. Repeat: "Ouch!" pain can be a life-saving signal and should *not* be endured. During exercise, feelings of muscle exertion for strengthening and stretch in the release of muscle tension and contraction are safe. "Ouch!" pain is a signal to *Stop!* Very often the exercise is dangerous and is the cause of the wrong muscle sensation, pain.

"Ouch!" pain rarely is caused by poor muscle tone or by your doing the exercise wrong. More than likely, such pain comes from an exercise that no one should do because it is impossible to do without "Ouch!" pain. Some excess discomfort or strong twinges may come from your doing an exercise that is too hard for your inadequately toned muscles, and sometimes pain can result from strain on already injured areas of the body such as a knee, shoulder, or the low back. In any case, if you feel "Ouch!" pain, *always stop!*

When teachers or coaches say, "If it hurts, it's good

for you," they are *wrong.* This traditional statement causes two harmful results. One obvious result is that injury often occurs if you go on. The other result is that many people carry this painful physical memory of exercise into adult life from school-time experiences and they hate exercise of any kind. People then feel "You're damned if you do exercise, and you're damned if you don't exercise." Exercise should not make you sore and aching; and if done correctly, should be satisfying enough in itself to stimulate continuing exercise. The correct exercises in the main part of this book should produce little lasting soreness and achiness in your muscles. And they are so beneficial and satisfying to do that they should stimulate you to continue to use them. They work — that is, they produce identifiable results that you can see and feel.

A further word about pain: Some exercises do not feel painful at the moment of doing them. The pain or injury from these can surface one or two days later. For example, bouncing, swinging, and fast exercises often cause the day-after soreness. This type of soreness can be prevented by not bouncing, swinging, or doing fast exercises. Another kind of pain can come about from a fall, a sudden and unexpected move, or an exceptionally heavy lifting or carrying maneuver. These types of injuries are harder to prevent but their pain can be minimized if proper warm-up and cool-down exercises are done. Toned muscles will also be less vulnerable to unexpected moves and recover more quickly because they are in better shape to begin with.

Strengthen the muscles you stretch.
Neither daily activities nor strenuous exercise (like running, jogging, swimming, biking, squash, and handball) provide muscles with a full balance of stretching and

strengthening maneuvers. Most strenuous activities strengthen the leg muscles and some aerobic activities strengthen the arms as well. In these activities as well as in daily activities, the abdominal muscles are often in a stretched or semi-stretched position. So it is crucial to strengthen the abdominal muscles properly. Some of the useless exercises people commonly do, such as side stretches, are supposedly for slimming the waistline. Side stretches actually stretch the side abdominal muscles. Correctly done curl-downs (the safe and effective substitute for fast one-direction sit-ups, see page 52), especially to each side, are very necessary to strengthen the stretched muscles. Inadequately strengthened abdominal muscles are one of the major reasons why back injuries are so common.

Stretch the muscles you strengthen.
A major cause of injuries to knees, ankles, elbows, necks, and the groin area is inadequately stretched

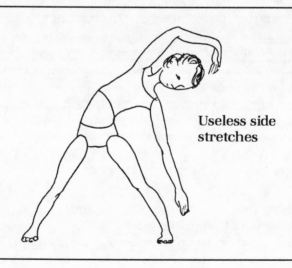

Useless side stretches

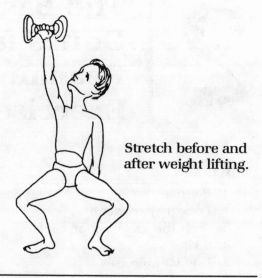

Stretch before and after weight lifting.

muscles. Some sports people never even bother to stretch their muscles. Those who do stretch may still use bouncing, which is both ineffective and a major cause of soreness to muscles (more about that on page 15, in chapter 2). The increasingly popular weight-training craze is inviting joint injury for many people because few weight lifters realize how important it is to stretch their muscles before and after lifting weights (see pages 38–40). The main part of this book contains safe and effective arm and leg stretches that will help prevent injuries to the major joints in the body.

2 | The Basic Don'ts for Readiness Exercises

Don't:

1. Bounce
2. Lock (hyperextend)
3. Arch the low back or neck
4. Swing
5. Do fast exercises
6. "Overbend" a joint
7. Click or pop

To ready your body for strenuous activity — dancing of any kind, skiing, skating, biking, any physically vigorous activity — you need to prepare your muscles, to stretch tight ones and strengthen weak or untoned ones. Once your muscles have been readied you can do any activity. Time spent in doing readiness exercises, sometimes called warm-ups, needs to be worthwhile. Exercises should be useful and safe. Any preparatory exercise that locks, bounces, swings, arches your neck or low back, is fast, or overbends a joint is harmful, useless, or both.

A word about the word *warm-up*, which literally means to raise the body's core temperature from its resting level. Any number of activities done for 30 seconds to a minute can raise the core temperature. Pushing against the wall for 30 seconds can warm the entire body. Running softly in place for 30 seconds to a minute can also. The best warm-up exercises to do are the simplest, like

14

pushing against a wall or walking around briskly. Readiness exercises are more than a warm-up and do more than just raise the core temperature; they prepare your muscles for activity. Neither warm-up activity nor readiness exercise should cause injury.

Here is why these six don'ts are to be avoided in exercises which you use to get ready for physical activity.

1. Do not bounce

Any time you are instructed to bounce, **Do Not!**

Bouncing, or pulsing, as some people say, does not effectively stretch or ready muscles for activity. The movement pathway of bouncing is one of up and down. The down part of the bounce does stretch a little, but then to carry out the command of "up," the muscles contract. Half of the bounce is a contraction, so 50 percent of the supposed stretch is *not* stretching! The continuous yes-no command, "stretch–don't stretch," that this down-up movement gives to the muscles can actually tear a muscle fiber. Bouncing is one of the major causes of soreness in your muscles because it tears the connective tissue web

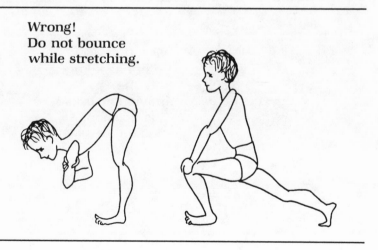

Wrong!
Do not bounce
while stretching.

that holds muscles together. Not only is this painful in itself, but it also causes fluid to come into the muscle, producing the tightness or slightly swollen sensation that you feel the next day.

2. Do not lock (hyperextend)

The joints most often locked are the knee and elbow. These joints are structured for mobility, not stability. Locking these joints gives a false sense of stability and strength to the limbs, and this encourages you to use your limbs in ways that place excess stress on these joints' binding structures. Strong sets of ligaments hold the bones together at these joints. Tendons of the arm muscles pass the elbow and tendons of the leg muscles pass the knee; and these tendons attach on or near the elbow and knee. The contraction and relaxation of the arm and leg muscles move the bones at the knee and el-bow joints, but the binding structure of these joints con-sists primarily of ligaments. That means, when you lock you are putting too much stress on the ligaments in

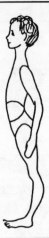

Wrong!
Do not lock knees.
Note the
arched low back.
This position
should be avoided.

these joints. Remember, ligaments don't have the power to shorten and lengthen the way muscles do.

When knees are locked (hyperextended), the bones in the joint press together in a way that often feels similar to gritting your teeth. Excess pressure in the joint can seriously damage the cartilaginous pads that are between the leg bones. Locking the knee also transfers the weight-bearing action from the thigh bone and muscles to the knee joint. The stretching and strengthening activity stops when the joint is locked, because there are only ligaments at the knee, *no muscles*!

Whether you have tight, loose, or average ligaments, you can and should learn to extend (straighten) your leg or arm without locking your knee or elbow. To practice feeling this unlocking, just lock your knee or elbow, to feel the stressful sensation of your bones pressing together; then simply relax the joint, unlock it, but do not bend it. You can recognize when the grinding feeling stops. Always unlock. Never again follow any instructions to lock your knees or elbows, be it in karate, ballet, wrestling, or any other activity. Learn to fully extend your knees and elbows without locking them.

Because experts from many fields understand the term *lock* in different ways, they also disagree about whether it is harmful or useful. To physicians the word *lock* merely means to become immobile; to karate teachers and weight lifters it means to jam and hold; whereas dance teachers often insist that legs be rigidly hyperextended. But you can learn to feel the difference between holding your limb firmly straight and over-tensing it when it is up against its natural stopping point.

3. Do not arch the low back or neck

A few words about the structure of your back: Paul C. Williams, M.D., author of several books on back pain and treatment, likens the spine to a stack of hockey pucks (the vertebrae) separated by jelly doughnuts (the intervertebral discs). Because there are few pain-sensitive nerve endings in the discs or in some of the ligaments that run up the vertebral column, there may be no immediate sensation of pain during a back-arching exercise to signal the exerciser to STOP! Some experts believe that back arching can force some of the fluid in the discs to seep out and cause permanent harm to the discs. All activities involving forceful or weight-bearing back arching need to be stopped.

Back bends are a prime example of weight-bearing back arching. Back bends, or "bridges," are an integral part of yoga, gymnastics, and some parts of dance training. Athletic and sports warm-ups often include waist circles, which are an example of a forceful exercise that includes rapid bending backward at the waist. The people who advocate back arching believe that you limber and strengthen your back in this manner. Because the

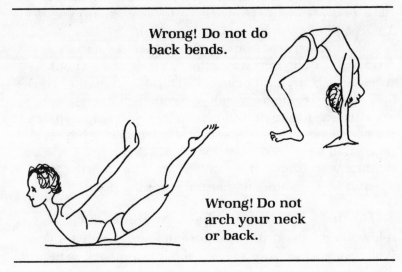

Wrong! Do not do back bends.

Wrong! Do not arch your neck or back.

Hockey pucks and jelly doughnuts: the structure of the spine — the vertebrae and discs

 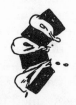

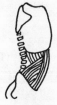

Three stomach muscles

case studies that show the harmful effects of back arching are not widely known, there is a debate among some experts about the dangers inherent in this exercise. And it is true that bodies are so varied in structure that some people experience the destructive results of back arching sooner than others. The anatomical information discussed above convinces me that any excess stress on the lumbar spine will sooner or later cause pain and eventually result in permanent damage.

Even your innocent morning stretch to take the kinks out of your awakening body needs to be carefully done so as not to arch too far backward. Just the standing position with your knees locked back causes a disc-squeezing excessive curve in the lumbar spine.

Many medical articles about the back start with the fact that 80 percent of doctor's visits are for low back pain. Why? There are two reasons, one of which is not often stated. Few people are aware that the human body is engineered with a major problem. The area in front of the lumbar spine (the low back) is only held in, up, and together with muscles. The second and well-known reason for so much back pain is that when the abdominal muscles are not adequately in tone, the lumbar spine has insufficient support. Then all the internal organs in front of the lumbar spine press against the lax abdominal muscles and strain the spine. Thus, to protect your low back, you need to stop all back arching and properly tone your abdominal muscles. (See curl-downs on page 53.)

Dropping your head backward can have a similar injurious effect on the discs in the neck part of your spine. Your head weighs 12–14 pounds. When that weight hangs back, passively, it puts pressure on the discs in the neck area of the spine and this pressure can begin to squeeze the fluid out of the discs. Continued excess squeezing can damage the discs and cause them to lose their hydraulic cushioning permanently. When the space between your discs is diminished, the muscles that attach to the vertebrae are being squeezed, causing dull, nagging pain. If the spaces are diminished even more, then nerves can be squeezed, causing sharp, "hot," shocking pain.

4. Do not swing

The swinging motion is used in exercises for legs and arms. Jumping jacks are an example of an exercise that uses arm swings. The swing occurs by means of momentum, and has most effect on the ligaments in the joint. Little or no muscle action occurs. But the outermost point of the swing can have the same effect on the muscles as a bounce can. In order for the limb to reverse direction there often is an abrupt and not very controlled stop, as in arm and waist swings from side to side. This abrupt reversal can tear muscle fibers and cause muscle soreness the next day.

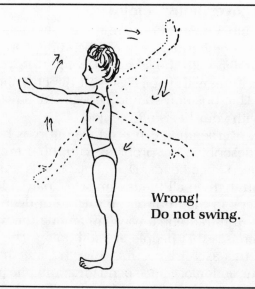

Wrong!
Do not swing.

5. Do not do fast exercises

Fast exercises for strengthening or stretching have the same harmful effects as swinging ones. Fast stretching exercises use momentum and can cause torn muscles when they require a sudden change of direction. Fast strengthening exercises cause the muscles involved to grab or suddenly bunch up. This doesn't strengthen the muscle correctly, but primarily tightens the already strong part of it in a jarring manner. Muscles that are strengthened by abrupt contraction gain very little ability to act in a slow and sustained manner. But when muscles are strengthened by slow and sustained training, they can easily be called upon to do fast, abrupt actions. Also, fast exercises such as fast sit-ups that are done to train weak muscles often cause "Ouch!" pain in the weak or injured area so they hurt the body more. Pain is always a signal to stop!

6. Do not "overbend" a joint

Your knees, elbows, and neck are the most vulnerable joints that can be injured from overbending. You are probably familiar with the severe discomfort in your knees after sitting with your legs bent directly underneath you. That position should be avoided. So should squatting with your heels off the floor.

The way overbending can produce injury is best explained by describing the problem with the exercise known as deep knee bends. Deep knee bends are intended to strengthen all the leg muscles, particularly the big quadriceps in the front of the thigh. But deep knee bends, done the traditional way, are among the most harmful exercises that people are still doing. The major problem in this exercise occurs when the knee bend is too deep. The action of a knee bend (or grand plié in dance) amounts to sitting down, buttocks toward the heels. When your legs bend and your upper body remains vertical, the initial loss of control and the beginning of the challenge to the thigh muscles occurs when your heels

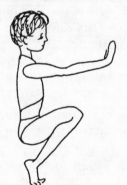

Wrong! Do not do deep knee bends.

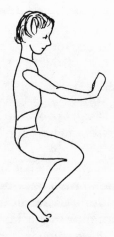

Safe, slow, controlled, not-too-deep knee bends

come off the ground. If the down and up action is done slowly *and* only to the place where your thigh muscles hold your body weight, this activity is beneficial and will increase your ankle, foot, and thigh strength. This corrected knee bend might be called slow, controlled, not-too-deep knee bends.

If the bend is too deep and goes beyond the place where the thigh muscles hold and control your body weight, or if your body just drops down, which happens when the exercise is done fast, then your knee ligaments suddenly and forcefully bear weight and can be very strained or even tear. Or the sudden forceful pressure can tear the cartilages and ligaments between the bottom of the thigh bone and the top of the leg bones. Football teams have successfully diminished the number of knee injuries of their players by eliminating deep knee bends, or "squat thrusts" that incorporate deep knee bends, from their training programs.

Your elbow can be injured in a similar manner when

doing pushups incorrectly. When you bend your elbows too much at the lowest point of the pushup, you've dropped below where your arm muscles hold and control your weight. In order to get up, you heave or throw yourself to lift your upper body back up, because your arm muscles are no longer directly controlling the action. Strained ligaments or muscles can result both from absorbing the sudden downward drop of the weight of your body and from the extreme effort required to heave your body back up. Overbending, like locking, is especially stressful in the knee and elbow because neither joint has any muscle. These joints are bound together by ligaments and only the tendons of muscles pass over them. The range of safe motion of your knee and elbow is limited to where arm and leg muscles control them and not beyond.

The neck part of your spine can be seriously injured when doing a shoulder stand. In a shoulder stand the neck is overbent forward (the opposite of arching). Neither the discs nor the vertebrae are structured to bear that much weight by themselves in that position.

7. Do not click or pop

Specialists disagree about what causes this click or pop sound and accompanying feeling of muscles or tendons rearranging. Preventing the click or pop is, however, important! Repeated clicking or popping can cause joint irritation. This sensation can happen in almost any joint: neck, shoulder, hip socket, knee, or ankle. Whenever you are doing any exercise or getting into a position to start one, do not let the click or pop occur.

You can prevent these sensations by slowing down your exercise; or by slowly rearranging your joint to start with, such as lowering your shoulder or centering your neck, or positioning your body weight more centrally over the entire surface of both your feet and pressing your toes. The important guideline to follow is to rearrange your joint, carefully and slowly, by moving it a little, usually into correct alignment (see page 91) and deliberately preventing clicking or popping in any of your joints.

Why These Harmful Activities Are Still Being Practiced

Tevye in *Fiddler on the Roof* bemoaned "tradition" to explain why today's habits are still practiced. Well, tradition appears to be the only plausible explanation for the continued use of bouncing, swinging, locking, arching, and fast exercises when research from many sources has demonstrated that these practices are useless or harmful or both. Human beings are "creatures of habit" and "habits die hard," so even if a coach or teacher has read about the harm of bouncing, for instance, he or she may forget to incorporate new and better techniques into the daily practice sessions simply because the system has become routine. All the information just summarized in this "Don'ts in Exercise" section is in books, easily available, and is taught in introductory courses for physical education teachers. None of this information is startling, new, or controversial.

Some of the exercise systems used today — in yoga, gymnastics, and ballet, for example — come from very old traditions that have spiritual, religious, or prestigious status. These systems are rarely questioned and people who quit these activities are considered unworthy or simply unable to meet the rigorous standards and requirements. Actually, the people who stop these activities because of the pain they experience are *wise.* But the routines of exercise are then left mostly unchanged and unquestioned. You trustingly take up these activities, not knowing that there are potential risks in some of the basic movements. And when you experience pain, you feel embarrassed to say, "Ouch! That hurts me." You even feel that you are the cause of the pain because you aren't in shape or doing it right. That is backward. If the exercise causes "Ouch!" pain, the exercise is harmful and should not be done!

Often these common exercises injure the joints, cause spinal discs to degenerate, tear the muscles that they are supposedly toning, and do not provide a balance of stretching and strengthening. The next section of this book will survey the body from head to toe and point out the harmful and useless popular exercises. And then, for each part of the body, basic strengthening and stretching exercises that work are described. These useful exercises will provide a way to ready your body for any physical activity *safely.* Included are explanations of what to feel, where to feel it, what parts of your body to protect and why.

In the instructions for stretching, the phrase "30 seconds to a minute" appears. Remember, the goal for stretching your muscles is for you to feel the release of tension. This sometimes takes more than a minute and sometimes takes less. You need to adjust the stretching time to each part of your body. But do hold each stretch position for at least 30 seconds. In the instructions for strengthening, the term a *slow count* means as the seconds tick on a clock or as if saying "a thousand" before each number, such as, "a thousand one, a thousand two, a thousand three . . ."

3 | Your Neck

The back and sides of your neck need stretching, while the front needs strengthening. However, **do not do head rolls.** The stated purpose of head rolls is to relax the tightness in your neck. This is supposed to ease tension and soreness in the back of your neck and tone up your neck muscles for good head posture. Instructions often say to drop your head to the chest, roll your head over to the left shoulder, then roll your head back and stretch the chin to the ceiling, then roll your head to the right so your ear is over the right shoulder.

There are three basic problems with this exercise:

1. By rolling your head back you are arching your neck and possibly damaging the discs in the neck area of your spine. This was described in the section "Do Not Arch," page 17.

2. Any time rolling or swinging is part of an exercise as in this head-rolling exercise, little or no toning or stretching actually occurs. Rolls and swings are passive and use momentum to maintain their motion.

3. The back part of head rolls increases the stretch of the muscles in the front of the neck, which don't need stretching, and contracts the back muscles of the neck, which are already too tight.

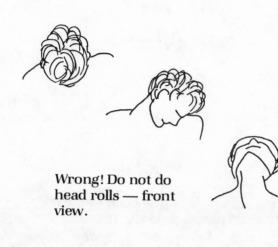

Wrong! Do not do
head rolls — front
view.

Wrong! Do not do
head rolls — side
view.

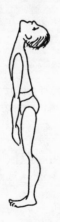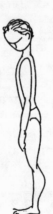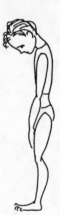

Do not do shoulder stands

This position is used in yoga and in an exercise called "the Bicycle." The problem for the neck in this position was described at the end of "Do Not 'Overbend' a Joint," page 21. Bearing your body's weight on your neck in this position puts excess pressure on the discs and on the bones. When you keep your chin straight forward on your chest, the neck discs are under such severe pressure that there is serious risk of causing a so-called "slipped disc," where the soft center part of the disc suddenly pushes through its outer case. The injury to the bones is more gradual. When bones are irritated, in

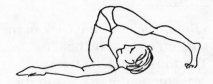

Wrong! Do not do the plow in yoga.

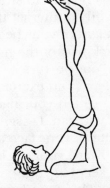

Wrong! Do not do a shoulder stand.

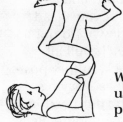

Wrong! Do not use the bicycle position.

this case by bearing weight in a manner they are not meant to do, the body's response to the irritation is to send calcium to the area; so the wear-and-tear type of arthritic calcium deposits can and do build up on those neck vertebrae. You may also feel light-headed after doing a shoulder stand because this position affects the blood supply to your brain and heart. The shoulder-stand position is also mistakenly used to stretch out the low back and even hamstrings, when it is not used for "bicycling." Safe ways to stretch hamstrings and low back are included in the back and thigh sections in this book, and do not put stress on the neck.

Correct Neck Stretches

But it *is* helpful to stretch the muscles at the back of the neck and counteract the tension caused by holding up the weight of your head. The muscles along the spine in the back part of the neck are among the tightest in the body. Poor posture or "forward head" adds to this problem. Here is an exercise to stretch tight neck muscles.

Straighten your neck in a vertical line, stretching as tall as you can. Lessen the curve in the back of your neck. Relax your face and jaw and carefully move your chin toward your neck. Lower your head toward your chest, keeping your jaw relaxed, your mouth open slightly. Place one hand on the top back of your head and gently pull your head forward and down. Do not let your chin touch your chest. Feel the stretch pull all along the muscles of the back of your neck. In that position, move your head a little to each side as if saying "No," holding each tipped position. Keep your head in each position and hold for 30 seconds to a minute. Relax your jaw. The pull of your hand is gentle.

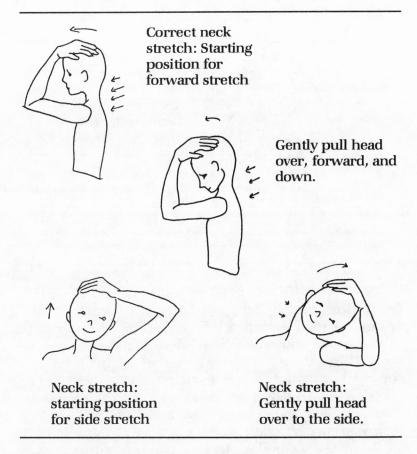

Correct neck stretch: Starting position for forward stretch

Gently pull head over, forward, and down.

Neck stretch: starting position for side stretch

Neck stretch: Gently pull head over to the side.

Return to a vertical position and curve your head sideways to the left, ear over your shoulder. Let your face stay looking forward, not down or up. Place your left hand on the right top side of your head and gently pull your head toward your left shoulder. Relax both shoulders and deliberately keep them down. Hold that position for 30 seconds to a minute. Keep your mouth and jaw relaxed, open, and loose. Repeat this gentle pull to the right side.

31

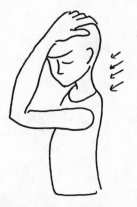

Neck stretch:
Gently pull head
diagonally forward.

Now return your head to the same position as for the first forward stretch and pull your head diagonally down toward the right, and then left. You will feel this stretch in the area of your neck where the back and side converge. This is the part of your neck that has not been stretched by the forward and side positions. These stretches can be felt in the muscles on both sides of the spine. Sometimes people feel this stretch as far down as their waists.

There is a method of stretching known as passive stretch that involves just hanging the head forward or to each side and allowing it to remain in that relaxed position. This method does not cause the soreness that bouncing and swinging do. The release of tension that results from passive stretch is minimal compared to actively, though gently, pulling on the head to stretch the neck muscles. The feeling of the active stretch is a relaxing sensation as the tightness of those muscles releases.

Correct Neck Strengthening

Head Raises

Head raises are for neck strength. Lie on your back, legs bent, knees up, and arms out to the sides, palms up, shoulders down.

1. Before beginning the head raises, lift your head one or two inches and stretch your neck longer, then lower your head to the floor; relax your jaw. Now lift your head slowly, starting with your forehead. Bring your chin up toward your chest. Take four slow counts to do this. Lower your head back to the floor, one vertebra of your neck at a time, putting your head down last. Take four slow counts to do this. The path your head makes is curved, not straight.

Neck strengthening exercise: starting position of the head and back

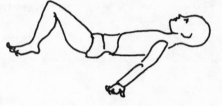

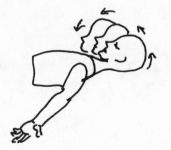

Neck strengthening exercise: Lift the head forward, chin toward the chest.

2. Now *turn* your head toward your right shoulder but do not move your head closer to your shoulder, just TURN your head. Lift your head slowly to bring your chin toward your shoulder. Take four slow counts. Lower your head slowly back down, putting your head down last. Take four slow counts.

3. Turn your head to your left shoulder. Repeat the lifting and lowering the same way as for the right. Take four slow counts up and four slow counts down. Take care to place your neck down toward the floor first and *not* your head.

Repeat this center, right side, left side, sequence two more times.

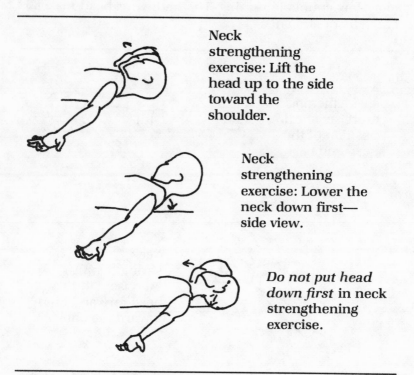

Neck strengthening exercise: Lift the head up to the side toward the shoulder.

Neck strengthening exercise: Lower the neck down first— side view.

Do not put head down first in neck strengthening exercise.

4 Your Arms and Shoulders

You need to *stretch* the *front* of your shoulders and *strengthen* the *back* of your shoulders. Your arm muscles need a balance of strength and stretch. **Do not do fast arm swings** to reach these goals. Fast arm circles, swings, and flings are often used to loosen the tight muscles in the shoulder area. Supposedly these exercises help relax shoulder and neck tension. Directions often say to circle the arms in large vertical circles forward or backward; or horizontally with arms held out to each side. When they are done fast they are practically useless and can increase soreness in your shoulder muscles and in the top part of your back.

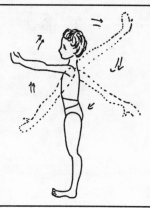

Wrong! Do not swing.

Correct Strengthening
for Arms and Shoulders

The first way to correct these exercises is to slow them down. Then the exercise becomes a strengthening one. Try one vertical arm circle to a slow count of 20: Take 10 counts to raise your arm in front of you from a starting position where your arm is hanging down at your side to above your head and 10 counts to complete the circle as you lower it down behind your body to the starting position. Imagine that your arm is cutting through cheese. This image lets you feel all the muscles of your arm in action. Repeat this circle 4–6 times. Now feel the warmth in your muscles! They are fatigued from this slow contracting action. When muscles are fatigued in this manner, the tightness does let go partially and relaxes.

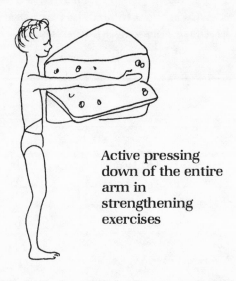

Active pressing down of the entire arm in strengthening exercises

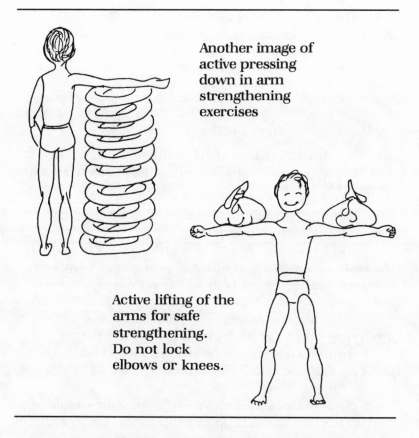

Another image of active pressing down in arm strengthening exercises

Active lifting of the arms for safe strengthening. Do not lock elbows or knees.

Try horizontal circles, your arms held out to each side to the same slow count, repeated 4–6 times. As you circle your arms, press down as though you were pressing a large spring and lift up as though you were lifting bags of sand. Take care to move only your arms at the shoulder, and hold your ribs, hips, and legs still.

Slow arm circles mildly strengthen the muscles that attach your arm to your shoulder. Fast arm circles can pull the ligaments in the shoulder excessively while not really stretching your shoulder muscles at all.

Pushups are a strengthening exercise commonly done for the arms and chest muscles. Pushups, too, are often done as fast as possible. Try them slowly and see how much more effective they are.

Pushups Corrected

Pushups should be done *slowly*, four slow counts down and four slow counts up. Several points of safety should be noted.

1. Your feet should be 2–4 inches apart and knees should be relaxed, not locked.
2. Your buttocks *should* be a little up, *out of line* with the rest of your body, in order to protect your low back. Stomach muscles must be held in and not be pushing out.
3. Your fingers should be spread and pressing the ground so undue strain is not felt in your wrists.
4. Your elbows should be neither locked when your arms are fully extended nor overbent when at the lowest part of the pushup.
5. Align your head straight out from your shoulders. Take care not to raise it up or drop it below a straight line. Relax your jaw; do not grit your teeth.

The number of pushups you do depends on your endurance. Your goal is to increase the number of repetitions — the speed should remain slow and constant. This is true for beginner pushups, done slowly leaning into and pushing away from a wall, as well as for horizontal ones with knees (or feet) on the floor.

For people using weights to increase arm and shoulder strength, three points are very important to remember:

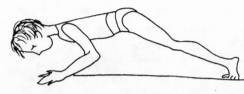

Pushup: lowered
position

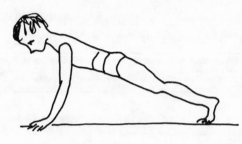

Pushup: raised
position

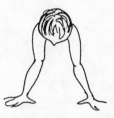

Wrong! Don't lock
your elbows in
pushups.

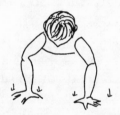

Press your fingers.

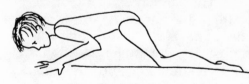

Position of the
beginner's pushup

1. Stretch your leg, arm, and shoulder muscles *before and after* weightlifting.

2. Do any and all weightlifting slowly in both directions, up 4–6 slow counts and down 4–6 slow counts.

3. Be sure to hold in your abdominal muscles. Whether sitting or standing, position your body so that you feel *no strain* in your low back. When standing, you can help to do this by keeping your knees slightly bent.

To prevent debilitating injury, it is much better to lift less weight for more *slow* repetitions than to lift too much weight a few times fast with excess strain on other very vulnerable parts of your body.

Correct Stretches for Arms and Shoulders

To stretch your shoulder muscles adequately, reach your arms behind your back, clasp your hands together, and lift your clasped hands and arms up. Whether sitting or standing, bend your head and chest forward so your arms can move higher. Tip one shoulder sideways and down so the other one is higher. You can feel a stronger stretch in the upper shoulder in this tipped position. Tip the other one up to repeat this increased stretch on the other side. Return your shoulders to a level position and lift your clasped hands higher. You should now feel a release of shoulder tension. This stretches your shoulder muscles from underneath. In the summary, this is called the underneath shoulder stretch. The two modifications of fast arm circles and this shoulder stretch illustrate the principle of balance between stretching and strengthening exercises.

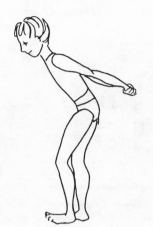

Starting position
for safe shoulder
stretch

Right shoulder up
in shoulder stretch

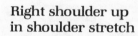

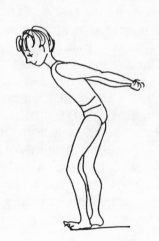

Lift both arms up
after stretching
one shoulder at a
time.

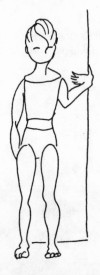

Safe shoulder muscle stretch from the side of the shoulder (side arm shoulder stretch)

There are two more stretches for the shoulder muscles, from the side, and from above, that help keep those muscles useful and flexible. These stretches feel good to do *before and after* running, biking, and swimming and even after writing, typing, and playing the piano.

To stretch the front of the shoulder area from the side, stand near a wall with your right arm extended at shoulder height and put your palm on the wall, fingers parallel to the floor and back. Unlock your elbow. Turn your entire body away from your arm, to the left and backward, then lean forward a little into the stretched shoulder. Hold this position 30 seconds to a minute. This stretch position even stretches the muscles in the forearm and wrist. Repeat this stretch with your left arm extended on the wall. In the summary, this is called the side arm shoulder stretch.

This next shoulder-muscle stretch works on these same muscles from above and requires a prop: a jump rope, or towel, or broomstick, or any piece of clothing that is at least 4–5 feet long. Sit down on the floor or on a chair. This sitting position protects your low back. Hold the rope with both arms outstretched, arms 3–4 feet apart. Carefully raise your extended arms above your head and back to the place that feels very tight on top of your shoulders. Hold the position at the tightest place. Be careful to keep your elbows unlocked and your neck and head vertical. Now shift that wide triangle to one side so that your right arm is almost above your head and your left arm is far out to the side. Relax the left

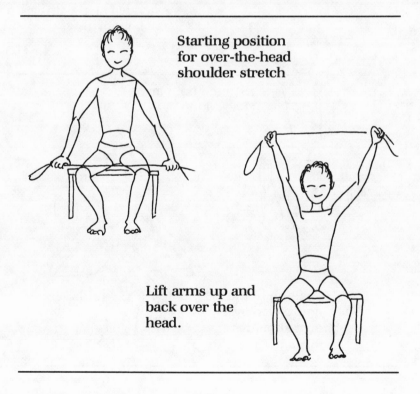

Starting position for over-the-head shoulder stretch

Lift arms up and back over the head.

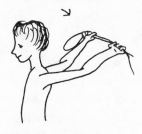

Side view of over-
arm shoulder
stretch

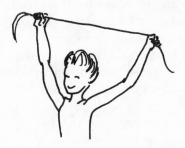

Stretch one
shoulder at a time
by pulling back the
extended arm with
the bent arm.

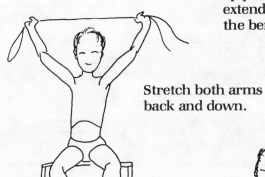

Stretch both arms
back and down.

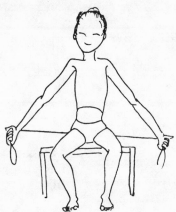

Position of the
completed over-
arm shoulder
stretch

elbow so that it bends and use the bent left arm to pull back gently on the right extended arm. This gentle pull will stretch the front of your right shoulder. Reverse this so that your left arm is up and your right arm is sideways and bent at the elbow. Let your right arm gently pull the left arm back and feel the stretch in the left shoulder. Now bring both arms back up above your head and try to take them both back behind you all the way without bending them, completing the arc so that your arms are down at your sides and the rope is behind you. If you can't do this now, widen the space on the jump rope. If this is too easy, close the space on the rope. Carefully bring the rope back up over your head and repeat this stretch over the top and back, once more. In the summary, this is called the overarm shoulder stretch. Remember to do these three stretches, from below, from the side, and from above, before and after any arm strengthening activity. Never do any of these stretches fast.

5

Your Back, Waist, and Stomach Area

The abdominal muscles — stomach and waist area — need strengthening; the back needs forward curved stretches. However, **do not do waist circles.** The supposed purpose of waist circles is to limber and slim your waistline and reduce your rubber tire. With legs wide apart, hands on hips, you are instructed to round the head and chest forward, then bend to the side, back, and side; or standing upright, twist from side to side. You are urged to do this fast. Why not? Four reasons:

1. Waist circles are similar to head circles in their harmful effects on the low back, the lumbar area of the spine. The backward position is dangerous to the discs of the low back because the weight of the upper body, pulling backward, puts excess pressure on the discs.

2. The backward pull also stretches the abdominal muscles, which are likely to be overstretched already because of the human upright position and because of passive habits of sitting, standing, and moving.

3. When the upper body is forward during this exercise, unless the abdominal muscles are strong already and held in, all the internal organs of this area put weight on the lumbar spine from the inside.

4. The side bend of waist circles stretches the criss-crossing set of stomach muscles at the waist; and so,

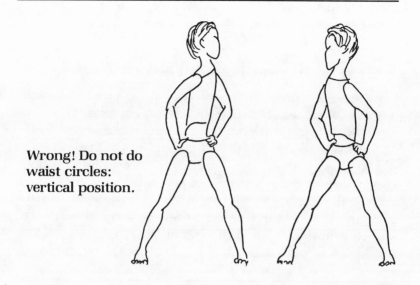

Wrong! Do not do
waist circles:
vertical position.

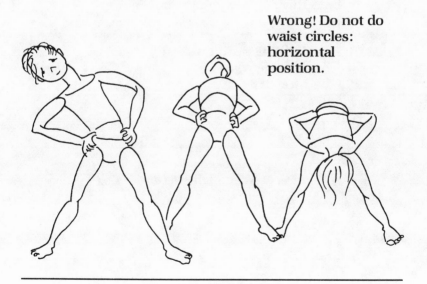

Wrong! Do not do
waist circles:
horizontal
position.

contrary to expectation, waist circles do not slim your waistline at all.

Safe Waist and Back Stretches

For a safe side stretch that does not stretch your stomach muscles but does stretch your lazy rib cage muscles, stand with feet 4–6 inches apart. Reach your arms to the ceiling; feel the stretching on the sides of your ribs and in the back along the spine. Bend your knees a little to help keep your buttocks slightly tucked under so there is no arch in the lumbar area of your back. Next, reach both your arms up and to one side, keeping your stomach flat and your buttocks down. Stretch up and to the other side. Hold each of these positions for 30 seconds to a minute.

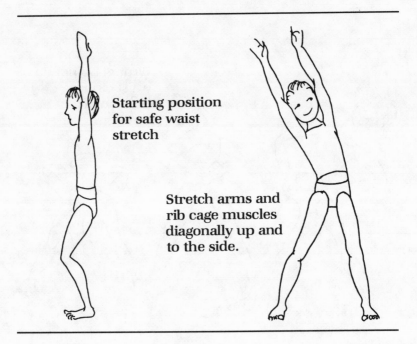

Starting position for safe waist stretch

Stretch arms and rib cage muscles diagonally up and to the side.

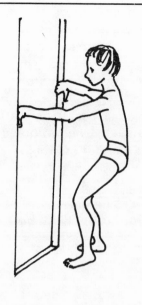

Pull back from
door frame.

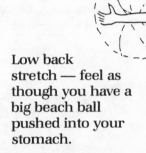

Low back
stretch — feel as
though you have a
big beach ball
pushed into your
stomach.

Last, hold your stomach in as if it could touch your
backbone. Bend your knees and let your arms come forward as though you had a very big beach ball pushed
into your stomach. Or, this position can be done by
holding on to the sides of a door frame and pulling back
against it, keeping your ribs and hips vertical and your
knees and shoulders forward. Feel this stretch along a
vertical line from the inside of the hipbone going up to
the ribs. If you feel no stretching sensation, then round
your head over a little, push your knees forward a little
more, tuck under and tighten your buttocks a little.

Do not do any type of back bend.

In yoga, gymnastics, and many types of dance classes, people are told to arch the low back in a variety of exercises and tricks. In the "**Don'ts** of Exercise" section, the reasons for not arching the low back and neck were discussed in detail. There is no correct or safe way to arch the back. Simply don't do it as part of an exercise routine or activity. (Sometimes passive back extension is used by physical therapists to help some back conditions. These rehabilitative exercises are not forceful or weight bearing. They are used for a limited number of physical problems.)

Some exercise systems use what is called the "prone arch," in which you lie stomach down on the floor, and

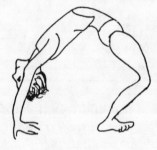

Wrong! Do not do back bends.

Wrong! Do not do the prone arch.

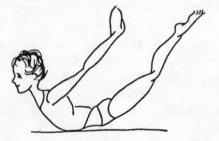

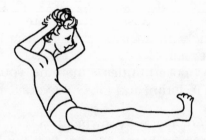

Wrong! Do not do sit-ups fast, or straight-legged, or with feet hooked under something, or with arms behind the head.

with arms behind your head, you lift first your chest, then your legs, so both the upper and lower halves of your body are off the floor. This squeezes the discs of the lumbar spine and stretches the abdominal muscles. It also is an exercise NEVER to do.

Do not do sit-ups: (1) fast, or (2) straight-legged, or (3) with feet hooked under something, or (4) with arms behind the head.

Sit-ups, the corrected version called curl-downs, can be very useful in strengthening abdominal muscles, thus improving posture and protecting the lower back. But if you are to benefit, you have to exercise those abdominal muscles without a lot of help from your arms or hips or from momentum of speed — and without arching your back.

1. Fast sit-ups with your legs straight and hands held behind your head do not properly tone the stomach muscles. Any exercise done quickly depends on momentum, not on muscle strength. Usually fast exercise also causes the muscles to grab, or suddenly to contract. Fast contractions build bulky muscles, so what tone does develop in the muscles is not pliable and not very useful.

2. When your legs are extended straight, the muscles on the top and side of your thighs, the hip flexors, do the work of lifting the torso. It is possible to lift your torso almost without using your abdominal muscles at all — and of course, it is easier.

3. When your feet are hooked under something, your feet assist the hip flexors in lifting and lowering your torso.

4. By placing your hands behind your head, you can use arm strength and a sudden heave forward to lift up from the floor. This too can be done without any use of your abdominal muscles.

Correct Curl-Downs for Abdominal Muscle Strength

Here is how to do sit-ups, now called curl-downs, correctly. Sit with your knees very bent and your chin tucked toward your chest. Hold your arms forward or place them on your chest. The goal is to keep them passive and not let them help lift your torso. Pull in the middle abdominal muscle and *hold it in* during the entire exercise. This is important. Many pictures show the middle muscle bulged out; the muscle is grabbing when it is out. Grabbing is a held, sudden contraction that does not allow the muscle to contract slowly and continuously all along its length.

Slowly roll backward down toward the floor, one vertebra at a time. The first part of this backward-rolling-down action is difficult because the bottom part of the spine does not bend. Keep the upper part of your body curved forward and progressively transfer your weight from the sit bones to the fleshy part of your buttocks. Keep your legs bent and actually move your feet nearer

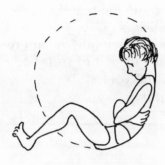

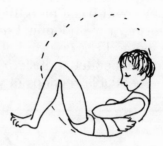

Center starting
position for
curl-downs

Lowest position for
center curl-downs

your body. Do not hold your feet down in one place on
the floor and do not extend the legs out into a straight
line.

Uncurl the spine down to the floor to about the middle of your rib cage; keep your chin tucked in and on
your chest, and you must at no time let the middle abdominal muscle push out. Now, without uncurling the
spine completely to lie flat on the floor, slowly return to
your starting position by curling up, leading with your
forehead, curving your head forward.

Imagine the uncurl and curl sequence taking place
inside the letter "O." Go down and come up slowly along
the same round pathway. Take 5–6 slow counts to go
down and 5–6 slow counts to come up. Do not stop between the down and up directions but keep the motion
smooth and slow. If 5–6 counts are too many, start with
3–4 and gradually take longer to go down and then up,
as you gain strength.

It is important to avoid opening at the hip joint like a hinge unfolding. When this joint is used incorrectly, the abdominal muscles only stabilize the torso and the movement has a path that looks like a "V" opening and closing. The abdominal muscles can actually remain re-laxed and not be taxed at all if the weight of your body is not deliberately transferred back off your sit bones onto the bendable sections of your spine.

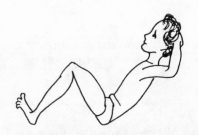

Wrong! Do not do curl-downs in a "V" position.

Doing the curl-downs back and forward is only the beginning. This slow uncurling down and curling up movement also needs to be done to each side. In the bent-knee, curved-back sitting position, rock to the right so that all of your body weight is on one buttock. Tip your entire body to the right, turn your head to the right, chin near your right shoulder, and look down to the floor over your right shoulder. Uncurl so that the side of your waistline presses on the floor. Continue to uncurl until your right shoulder is on the floor, or near it. Curl up, keeping your head and neck relaxed but out over the floor, and retrace the pathway used going down. Make sure to *hold in* your middle abdominal muscle. Keep your legs bent and tipped to the right. Now repeat this sequence on the left side.

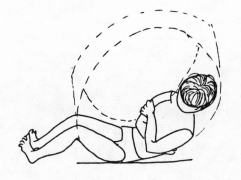

Starting position for curl-downs to the side

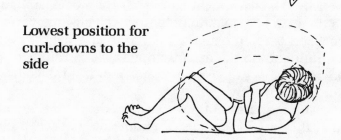

Lowest position for curl-downs to the side

Uncurl down and curl up to the center, to the right side, and to the left side, three times over. Each curl sequence takes 5–6 counts down and 5–6 counts up. This is the best exercise to build and maintain abdominal muscle strength and therefore to protect your low back. If during any part of this sequence your middle muscle pushes out, either carefully pull it in, or come up enough to pull it in, and continue the sequence. If necessary, come up to start again, but do not practice the mistake of doing curl-downs with the middle muscle bulging out. Do not jerk your body during any part of this exercise.

Do not do double leg lifts.

Double leg lifts require you, while lying on your back, to lift both your legs up straight, to a right angle from the floor, and then to lower them, fast or slowly. This difficult and uncomfortable exercise is supposed to strengthen your stomach muscles fast. But muscles do not build strength overnight. This exercise is a prime example of working with the wrong sets of muscles in ways that can do more harm than good. Very few people are able to do this strenuous exercise while keeping their low back area pressing flat on the floor during the entire activity. The leg weight causes a severe back arch, which is dangerous. While doing double leg lifts, many people feel sudden and extreme pain in their low backs but continue to do the exercise nonetheless. **Pain is a signal to stop!!** This exercise illustrates that **if it hurts, it is** *bad* **for you, so stop!**

The exercise routines that include double leg lifts say that they are for increasing abdominal muscle strength. Yet the major muscles that lift the legs during the first half of the distance from the floor are the hip flexors. Once the abdominal muscles get into the act, they are called upon for emergency work to prevent that back arch. This often means they will grab and push out, the opposite of what is beneficial!

As an exercise to strengthen abdominal muscles, double leg lifts are of little benefit. Curl-downs as described in the preceding section are the most beneficial exercise for your three abdominal muscles. Even modified leg raises, done one leg at a time, only mildly strengthen the legs and do little to flatten your stomach area. The abdominal muscles are working only to stabilize the body by holding the hips and ribs in alignment during the leg lifts.

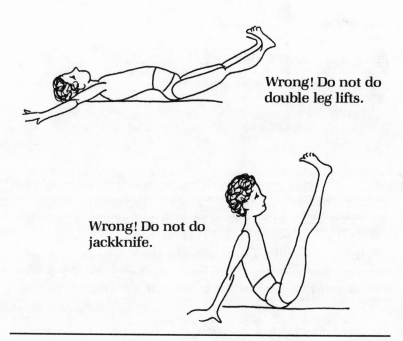

Wrong! Do not do double leg lifts.

Wrong! Do not do jackknife.

The "jackknife," with your weight supported on the buttocks and on the hands, is an upright version of double leg lifts. It causes strain to the low back similar to that just described. In addition, people feel severe strain to the discs in the rib area of the spine. This is another exercise you *should not do.*

6 | Your Legs

All leg muscles need stretching because most aerobic activity contracts and strengthens leg muscles. Legs are very important in all physical activity; yet many exercisers injure parts of their legs. There are many exercises for the legs: for the front, outside, back, and inner thigh, the calf, the ankle, and the foot; yet many people don't understand how crucial it is to do these exercises correctly.

Your Calf

In order to ready your legs for most physical activity, the first stretch to do is the calf stretch.

Do not bounce the calf stretch (or any other stretch!).

Correct stretching of your calf muscles — the muscles on the back of the lower leg — is very important to do **before and after** walking, running, hiking, swimming, or any other activity that uses your legs, because the calf muscle lifts your heel and pushes you forward. Not stretching the calf adequately or properly can lead to tendonitis at the ankle and to knee injury also.

Correct Calf Stretch

To stretch the calf muscle or any other muscle ade-

quately, you need to hold the stretching position for at
least 30 seconds; and of course a minute is even better.
To stretch the calf correctly, stand with your torso leaning forward, the upper body, head, chest, and stomach
all in line. Extend one leg back and bend the other leg.
Place the foot of the extended leg straight back, toes
straight forward, heel directly behind your toes. Relax the
knee of the reaching-back leg. Feel the weight of your
body over the front bent leg and keep that foot flat, heel
down. Now press your rear heel down and feel the
stretch all along your calf muscles.

By slightly bending the knee of the stretching leg, you
can feel the stretch move lower or higher in your calf
muscle. Once you actually feel the stretch in your calf
muscles, then you can use the position of leaning against
the wall that is often shown in instructions for the calf
stretch. You need to adjust the position in order to make
it useful. The wall calf stretch is safe: If you place your
feet far from the wall, 2–3 feet; if you actually feel the

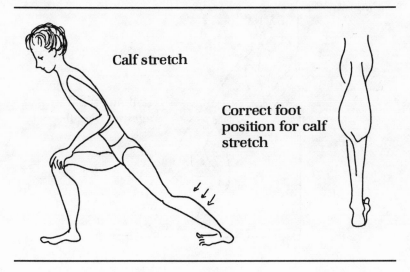

Calf stretch

**Correct foot
position for calf
stretch**

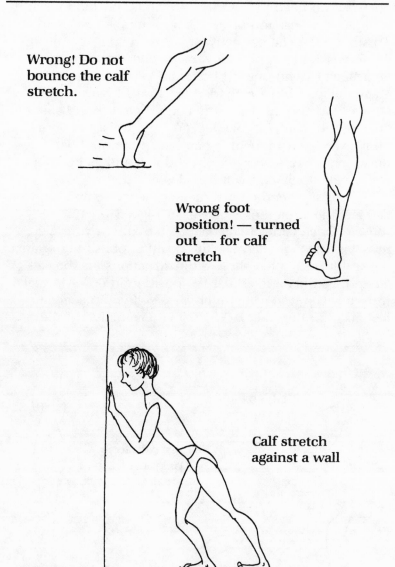

Wrong! Do not bounce the calf stretch.

Wrong foot position! — turned out — for calf stretch

Calf stretch against a wall

stretch in your calves; if your knees remain relaxed; if your chest and head remain forward; and if you hold your stomach in to protect your low back. Do not push away from the wall but do lean on it. Of course, do not bounce. If you stretch one leg and then the other, instead of two at once, the discomfort of the initial tightness in the muscle is easier to tolerate and let relax.

When this stretch is done by just holding the calf muscle in a position that adequately stretches the muscle, the feeling of tightness changes to a feeling of released tension. Tightness in the muscle lessens and your muscle relaxes. It is important to let this happen and to become sensitive to this releasing sensation. You feel the lengthening and see the proof because the bend at your ankle increases.

The Back of Your Thigh

Once you have stretched your calves, then stretching the other parts of your legs — all the sides of your thigh — is much more comfortable.

Do not do traditional toe touching.

Toe touching is an old standby in every exercise system. It is intended to stretch the hamstrings, the muscles located along the back of the thigh. Pictures show knees locked, and instructions say to bounce, or lift and lower the arms and torso until your hands can touch your toes or the floor. But when knees are locked, there is damaging strain on the knee joint.

Often toe touching is prescribed as a way to slim the waistline. It is a mistake to suppose that this exercise benefits your abdominal muscles or your waistline. During this exercise, the body bends at the hips, not the waist, so the waist area is not even actively bending. If

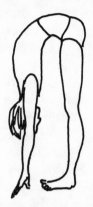

Wrong! Do not do traditional toe touching.

done with the abdominal muscles relaxed, toe touching can cause or increase pain in the area of the lumbar spine because the internal organs are pressing on the abdominal wall and pulling the lumbar spine into an arch on the way down and up.

Correct Hamstring Stretch

Here is how to get the most out of this hamstring stretch. Before you bend your upper body down:

1. Place your feet 4–6 inches apart and straight forward.
2. Hold in your stomach, stand tall and relax your jaw.
3. Bend your knees a lot.

Now, bend your upper body at the place where your legs join your hip sockets, and fold yourself down so your upper body touches your thighs and your palms are on the floor in front of your feet. Bend your knees as much as needed in order to do this; this bent leg and folded position protects your low back, as does holding your stomach firm. If the backs of your thighs are so tight that your body is almost in a squatting position, place a telephone book or two under your palms. Keep your elbows relaxed and don't push up from the floor. If you feel pain in your calf muscles or behind your knees, then place a telephone book (1–2 inches thick) under your heels to do the following stretch sequence.

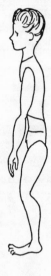

Safe hamstring stretch: starting position for lowering upper body

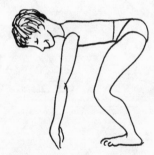

Going down into the safe hamstring stretch

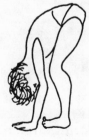

Starting position for hamstring stretch

Now work on the leg stretch by partially straightening one leg and holding it semistraight for 6–10 counts. Keep your rib cage firmly touching the thigh that is straightening. Relax that first leg and straighten — but not to a locked position — the other leg, and hold that position for 6–10 counts. Keep your rib cage touching your thighs during the entire straightening process and aim your buttocks up to the ceiling. Do not straighten your legs entirely — and do not lock them — unless you can keep your upper body completely touching your thighs.

When both of your legs, one at a time, have been

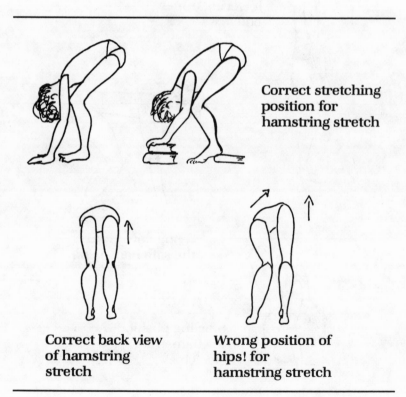

Correct stretching position for hamstring stretch

Correct back view of hamstring stretch

Wrong position of hips! for hamstring stretch

stretched twice, rock forward, transferring your body weight onto your palms, keeping your chest on your thighs, and then straighten both legs as far as is reasonable. Stay in this position for 6–10 counts; transfer your weight back to your feet, staying in the same hanging-down position; and transfer your weight forward once more onto your hands, straighten both legs again, with your chest on your thighs, and hold to feel more tension release in your hamstrings.

To stand upright, bend your knees and round your back. With your abdominal muscles held in, uncurl to a standing position. Only straighten your legs after your torso is vertical. This way of standing up and bending down protects your lumbar spine from strain and prevents very painful back trouble, which can be triggered by doing traditional toe touching.

Another version of this hamstring stretch involves placing one leg up on a park bench, the trunk of a car, or some other available raised surface where your foot can rest so that you can reach over and lean the upper body forward over that raised leg. If done correctly, this way of stretching the hamstrings is very effective.

When doing this stretch, first bend the knee of the lifted leg so that the hip, waist, and chest are touching the top of the thigh. **Hold abdominal muscles in!** Hug your leg by reaching both your arms around that thigh. Relax your head and jaw forward. Slowly work toward straightening the raised leg, keeping your hips and chest touching your thigh. The stretching sensation of the muscles along the back of your thigh is clearly felt in this process. You do not need to straighten your leg entirely to get a very good stretch-pull when doing this stretch in this manner. Stay 30 seconds to a minute in this position. Repeat this stretch with the other leg. Take three precautions:

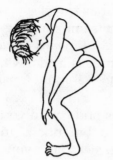

Safe coming up from hamstring stretch: starting position

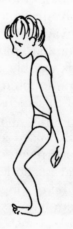

Keep knees bent while raising upper body.

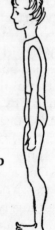

Finish standing up by straightening your legs.

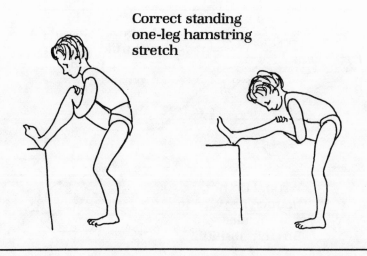

Correct standing
one-leg hamstring
stretch

1. Keep the knee of your hugged leg in an upright position, that is, do not rotate your leg out or in.

2. Keep your standing leg forward, with knee unlocked, and press your toes firmly on the ground for balance.

3. Keep your upper body against your thigh by folding forward where your thigh inserts into your hip.

Stretching the Front of Your Thigh

It is difficult to find a stretch for the big thigh muscle that does not make some other part of you uncomfortable. The "Hurdler's Stretch," a sitting stretch with one leg bent back, is often used for this, but it is risky.

Do not do the "Hurdler's Stretch" in the wrong position.

Used with extreme caution, the "Hurdler's Stretch"

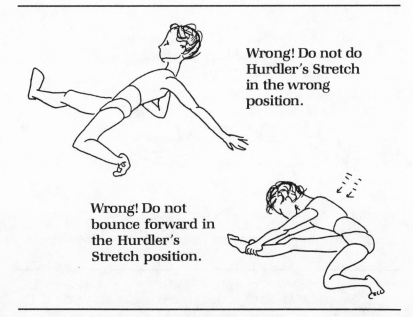

Wrong! Do not do Hurdler's Stretch in the wrong position.

Wrong! Do not bounce forward in the Hurdler's Stretch position.

position is useful for stretching the top of your thigh, your quadriceps muscles. If not done carefully, however, great strain is placed on the knee of the bent leg.

Correct Quadriceps Stretch

The "Hurdler's" position involves sitting with one leg bent, placed diagonally behind your body and turned over so the inner part of your thigh is on the ground. Your other leg is bent and in front of you. The position of the foot of the leg bent behind you is crucial in preventing injury to that knee. Your foot must not be kept at a right angle to your leg; it should be extended, pointing down along the line of your lower leg in a relaxed way, and not pointed forcefully. Don't twist your lower leg by turning your foot over. Bring your foot as close to your buttocks as is comfortable, not far away and not so close as to be almost sat on. Your other leg is bent to protect your lumbar spine from strain.

Now that you are sitting in the correct position, the next two moves will produce a stretch in the top of the thigh of your bent back leg.

1. Lean diagonally back, slowly and smoothly, onto the forearm and elbow opposite your bent back leg. Do not arch your low back. This position pulls your upper body diagonally down and back in line away from your bent back leg. Reach your other arm toward the knee of your bent front leg. Hold this position for 30 seconds to a minute.

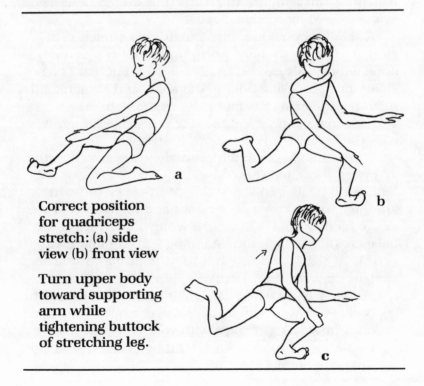

Correct position for quadriceps stretch: (a) side view (b) front view

Turn upper body toward supporting arm while tightening buttock of stretching leg.

2. Tighten your buttock muscles to lift the hip of your bent back leg up a little to increase the thigh stretch and turn your upper body toward the arm you are resting on. Hold that position for 30 seconds to a minute and then return to the first position. While you feel the tightness in your upper thigh release, you should not feel any strain in your knee, especially in the part of the knee near the floor. Repeat this stretch on the other side.

This position is often used to stretch the hamstrings as well, and pictures show the upper body rounded and bouncing forward over the extended leg. If you do it in this straining manner, you risk knee, groin, and back injury. Therefore, do *not* use this position to stretch the hamstring. Instead, use the hamstring stretch described in the preceding section, page 62.

A standing version of this quadriceps stretch is included in many runners' warm-up sequences, and if it is done wrong, this can be another knee cruncher. The position involves taking hold of the ankle and stretching the thigh by squeezing the foot close to the buttocks. Though some people feel the thigh muscles stretch this way, the knee joint is being overly strained.

To do this thigh stretch properly while standing, the following sequence should be done: Stand on your left foot, bend your right leg, and lift it up, knee **forward** and high. While using your right hand to grasp your right ankle, hold on to a wall or tree with your left hand for balance. Do not lock your standing leg. Carefully swing your bent right leg down and back, pointing your knee straight down to the floor. Push your right foot back against your hand while your right hand pulls your bent leg back. Push your foot away from your buttocks while making almost a right angle with your bent leg.

Do not squeeze your knee tight by pushing your heel toward your buttocks!!!

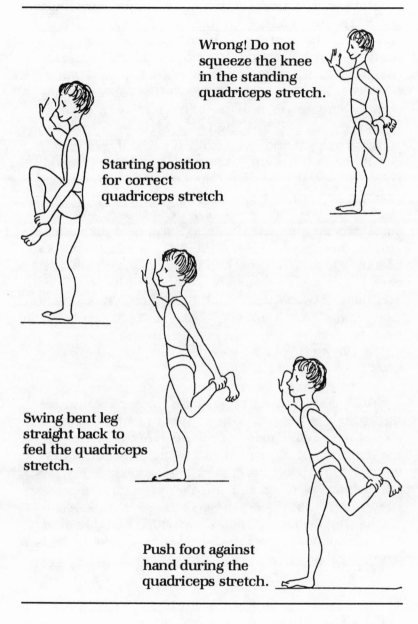

Wrong! Do not squeeze the knee in the standing quadriceps stretch.

Starting position for correct quadriceps stretch

Swing bent leg straight back to feel the quadriceps stretch.

Push foot against hand during the quadriceps stretch.

Hold your stomach in and do not arch your lumbar spine. Tip your chest forward to help prevent arching your back. The stretch feeling should be felt along the front of your thigh. Hold the position for 30 seconds to a minute or until the tightness releases. You should not feel any discomfort in your knee or just above it. If any pain is felt here, open the bend in your leg by giving more leg push and less hand pull. Make sure your knee is straight down and not slightly lifted to the side.

Here is another stretch for your quadriceps that involves no possible strain on the knee joint. Find a surface, flat and smooth, about as high as the middle of your thigh. The back of a sofa, a desk, the trunk end of some cars are possible surfaces. Stand near the surface and lift one bent leg up onto it. By pivoting on your supporting leg, turn your back to the surface. Or with your back to the surface, carefully lift one bent leg to the side and then slowly swing it back and up onto the surface. Hold your stomach in.

Do not arch your back while lifting your leg side or back!!!

Your bent leg is now resting on the surface and your upper body is forward. Take care not to arch your back. To feel the stretch, just rest the thigh of the bent leg on the surface in this position and tighten the buttock of that leg. Then bend the supporting leg, press down against your bent leg, and you should feel the thigh stretch. Your upper body remains forward, arms resting on the supporting leg. Hold the position for 30 seconds to a minute or until you feel the tightness release. Repeat with the other leg.

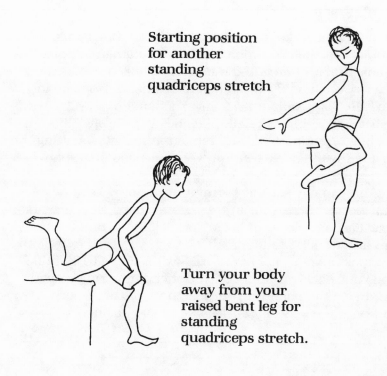

Starting position
for another
standing
quadriceps stretch

Turn your body
away from your
raised bent leg for
standing
quadriceps stretch.

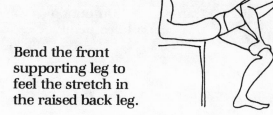

Bend the front
supporting leg to
feel the stretch in
the raised back leg.

Strengthening the Front of Your Thigh

Do not do deep knee bends! Traditionally deep knee bends have been recommended to strengthen the quadriceps, the front area of the thigh. A detailed explanation of why you should not do deep knee bends appears in the "Do Not 'Overbend' a Joint" section, on page 21. This instruction applies to daily activities that involve kneeling or squatting. Simply do not remain in a deep squatting position with your weight on your toes and knees, no matter what the reason.

You can correct this harmful position by keeping your heels on the floor in the manner used all across the Near East and Far East Asian countries, if your calf muscles and Achilles tendons (that attach your calf muscle to the back of your heel bone) are flexible enough. By putting your heels on the floor, you then support your body weight on the bones of your feet, horizontally placed, and on the bones of your legs, vertically positioned, in-

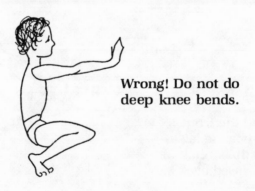

Wrong! Do not do deep knee bends.

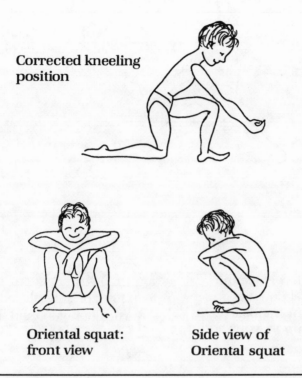

Corrected kneeling position

Oriental squat: front view

Side view of Oriental squat

stead of on your knee ligaments and cartilages with the bones of your legs precariously balanced on a diagonal.

Some martial arts, fencing, and dance exercises require a one-legged deep squat with the other leg extended to the side. This position strains the knee of the overbent leg and can produce an excessively strong stretch on the inner thigh of the extended leg. It can be made safe by placing the heel of the overbent leg down on the floor, as explained in the preceding paragraph. This position requires fairly stretched calf muscles and should not be attempted without first stretching the calf

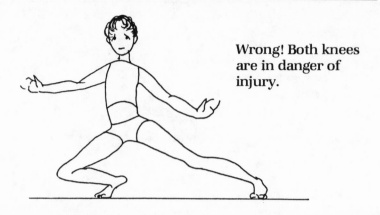

Wrong! Both knees are in danger of injury.

Safer: Place the heel down and use your hands to support your body.

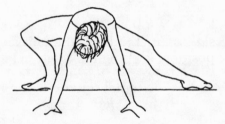

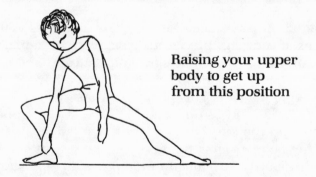

Raising your upper body to get up from this position

and hamstrings of both legs. Do not stay in this position if the heel of the bent leg is not down on the floor. Tip the upper body forward and toward the bent leg to maintain balance and enable you to rise.

Correct Quadriceps Strengthening Exercises

The following exercise is an adaptation of the one used to strengthen the quadriceps after a knee injury. If necessary, stand near a wall to hold and maintain balance. The standing leg should be relaxed, the knee unlocked, and the foot pointed straight ahead. Bend the other knee so that the lower leg is almost at a right angle to its own thigh. Lift that bent leg up, in front of you, about 6–8 inches. Slowly straighten the leg by extending the lower leg; do not lower the knee. Take care to raise the lower leg up, and take 6 slow counts to do this. Then take 6 slow counts to bend the lower leg back to the beginning position, keeping the thigh held at the first angle. Fully extend your leg, but do not lock your knee when your leg is straight.

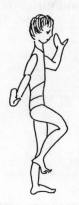

Starting position for quadriceps strengthening exercise

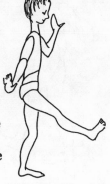

Slowly extend the raised leg for strengthening the quadriceps.

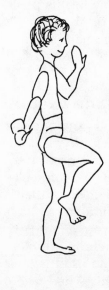

Raise the leg to continue the quadriceps strengthening exercise.

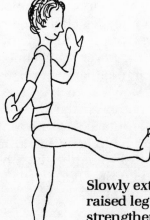

Slowly extend the raised leg again for strengthening the quadriceps.

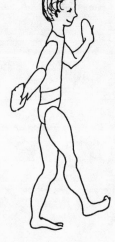

Slowly lower the raised leg to finish the quadriceps strengthening exercise.

Raise your thigh another two to three inches and repeat. Raise your thigh again, this time parallel to the floor, and extend your lower leg again. When this sequence is complete, slowly lower the extended leg to the floor, 6 slow counts.

Take care to hold your upper body in a vertical line and hold your stomach muscles in. You should not feel strain in the low back or the knee of the supporting leg. Repeat this sequence with your other leg. When you complete this exercise, do either of the quadriceps stretches, sitting or standing, page 68.

The following exercise is more strenuous than the preceding one and also builds strength in your thighs with minimal risk to the knees. Stand with one foot well ahead of the other, 10–14 inches apart. Slowly, take 6–8 counts to bend both knees; lower your body while keeping your upper body in an almost upright vertical position. Feel your body weight over your front leg. The heel of your back foot lifts up while the heel of the front foot remains on the ground during the entire exercise. When the knee of your back leg is almost on the ground (do not rest it down) then slowly, 6–8 counts, straighten your legs, raising your body up again. The front foot and leg should be positioned so that, at the lowest point, your thigh and lower leg are at a right angle. Repeat this two more times with your legs in this same position. Then place the back leg forward so that the exercise can be repeated for the other side. Repeat the down, up sequence, 6–8 counts down and 6–8 counts up, three times.

This exercise demonstrates how to feel the exertion of muscle-strengthening activity in a safe way. Be sure to feel the strengthening fatigue smoothly and continuously during the entire exercise. Make sure that you do not feel any discomfort in your knees. If you do feel knee discomfort, adjust the space between your legs, forward or

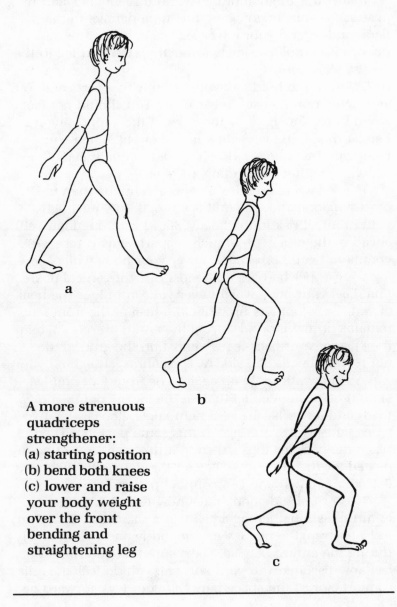

A more strenuous
quadriceps
strengthener:
(a) starting position
(b) bend both knees
(c) lower and raise
your body weight
over the front
bending and
straightening leg

back, and do not lower your body down quite so far.
When you have finished doing this strenuous exercise, it
is important to carefully stretch your calves, hamstrings,
and quadriceps, using the stretches listed for them.

Stretching the Upper Hip

One of the strongest and least stretched areas of the
body is your buttocks and the top backs of your thighs.
All leg activity tightens these muscles, and it is important
to stretch them. Here is how to stretch this area. The position is called "the Pretzel."

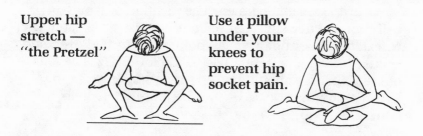

Upper hip
stretch —
"the Pretzel"

Use a pillow
under your
knees to
prevent hip
socket pain.

Start by sitting in a cross-legged position. Now put
your left leg, bent at the knee, flat on the floor so that
your left foot is near your buttocks and your left knee is
lined up in front of your belly button. Put your right leg,
very bent at the knee, over the left lower leg, in the same
way that your legs are positioned when you sit in a chair
with your legs crossed at the thighs. Your two knees are
nearly one above the other. Lean your upper body and
arms forward and hang your head down over your knees.
Bend your elbows and try to put your forearms down on
the floor. Feel this stretch on the sides of your thighs and
in the lower sides of your buttocks. Repeat with your legs
in reverse positions.

If sitting in this position is uncomfortable in the front of your hip sockets, put a 2–3 inch telephone book or pillow under your knees. If stretching forward is too uncomfortable at first, lean to the left and then to the right, using your left and then right hand and forearm to lean on, and hold for 30 seconds on each side. Then lean forward over both knees and hold for 30 seconds to a minute.

If your hips are so tight that you cannot bring your body forward, then lean on the floor to the side of the foot of the top leg. The stretch will be felt more in the thigh of the upper leg than in that of the lower. This stretch will be evened out when you repeat it with the legs in the reverse positions.

Guard against knee pain. The position of your feet will protect your knees. The foot of the lower leg should be extended but not strongly pointed or turned over, and should not be at a right angle to the lower leg. The foot of the upper leg should be kept at a right angle to the lower leg but not sickled — not bent at the ankle to either the left or the right.

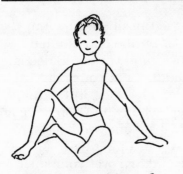

Starting position of "the Pretzel": lower leg position

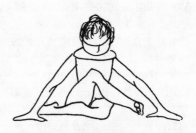

Starting position of "the Pretzel": upper leg position

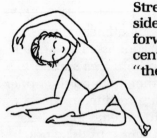 Stretch to each side before leaning forward into the center position of "the Pretzel."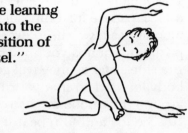

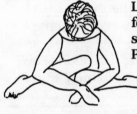 Lean upper body forward to feel the stretch of "the Pretzel" position.

Partial stretch for one hip, then the other for "the Pretzel"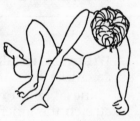

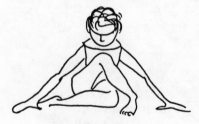 Wrong foot position! for "the Pretzel"

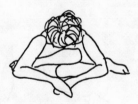 Deep Pretzel stretch

Your Inner Thigh

This area requires careful stretching. However, **Do not do the "Japanese (or Chinese) Split,"** sometimes recommended as a warm-up exercise for runners. This stretch position requires you to stand with both legs spread to the side as far as they will go, and then to bend the upper body forward so that your hands are resting on the ground. Instructions say to hold this stretch for at least 10 seconds and to repeat it several times. In this stretch there are two serious risks, one to the knees and the other to the muscles and tendons of the inner thigh. This stretch produces a very strong pull on the entire groin area. The strength of the stretch is likely to produce pain, not just a strong stretching sensation. The body's automatic response to pain is to tighten, to con-

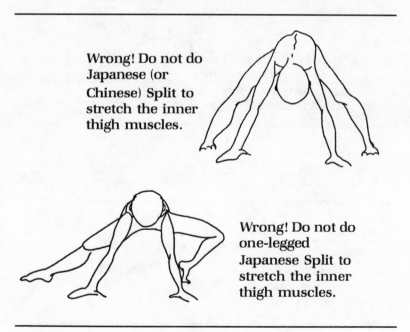

Wrong! Do not do Japanese (or Chinese) Split to stretch the inner thigh muscles.

Wrong! Do not do one-legged Japanese Split to stretch the inner thigh muscles.

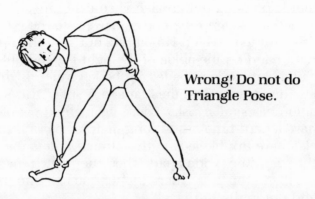

Wrong! Do not do Triangle Pose.

tract against the pain, as though to pull away. While in this stretching position, there is a great deal of the body weight pulling down on those tight muscles. The very muscles you want to relax are very likely to do the opposite, and the result is a possible tear. Furthermore, the knees are in their most vulnerable position because they are not meant or able to bend sideways, only backward and into a straight position; and even a slight bend, sudden or not, in response to recovering from the extreme stretched position or in response to the extreme discomfort of the position, could easily cause a strained ligament or a torn cartilage. This is one of those warm-up positions that cause injury or make players' legs, in football, track, or soccer, more susceptible to injury. There are better, safer, and more comfortable ways to stretch the inner thigh muscles, as will be described later in this section.

A standing yoga position, often called the "Triangle Pose," also invites this same groin injury. This position is often used for inner-thigh stretching in soccer, track, and football. The "Triangle Pose" has the exerciser stand, legs

wide apart, arms stretched out to the sides. The right
foot is pointing out, the left is straight forward. Now, instructions say, tip the body sideways to the right toward
the right foot, which is pointing out; and then place the
right hand on the ankle of the right leg and hold that position. Stretch is to be felt in the left inner thigh. Though
less dangerous than the "Japanese Split," this stretch position has similar risks. Loose-ligamented people will
have a hard time not locking their knees, and they may
also have trouble feeling this stretch unless they place
their legs very wide apart. Then the stretch may be felt
mostly in the area where the tendons go into the groin
and not in the muscles.

Correct Inner-Thigh Stretch

Flexible inner-thigh muscles allow your legs to reach easily in all directions, which is necessary in activities like
tennis, soccer, and karate. The following stretch helps to
provide this range of motion. Sit on the floor and place
the bottoms of your feet together, knees out to each side.
Do *not* pull your feet in toward your hips but place them
in a comfortable position where they fall naturally, making a diamond shape. Put your hands on the floor 5–10
inches behind your hips, rock your legs to the right so
that your right leg is on the floor, and lift your hips off the
floor, tipping your hipbone back to straighten your spine.
Let the weight of your left leg pull down to the floor. Hold
this position for 30 seconds to a minute. Sit down and
rock your legs to the left so that your left leg is on the
floor. Repeat the hip lift, and let the weight of your right
leg pull down to the floor. Hold this for 30 seconds to a
minute. Now, let your right leg pull your legs into an even
position so both knees are at an equal distance from the
floor. Let the bottoms of your feet fall open, and imagine

that you have a weight on each knee. Hold this position for 30 seconds to a minute more. You will feel this stretch along the upper inner-thigh area below the groin. Sit down and pull your body forward by placing your hands on your ankles and pulling your head down toward your feet. Put your elbows out to each side. Bend your body forward at the place where your thighs go into your hip-bone, not at the waist, and be sure to keep the weight of your body on your entire buttocks, not forward of them. Hold that pulled-down position for 30 seconds. You will feel this part of the stretch along the entire length of your inner thighs and sometimes on the underside of your thighs as well. Repeat the hip lift position again, rocking your legs first to one side and then to the other. Sit back down on the floor and repeat the pulling-forward position.

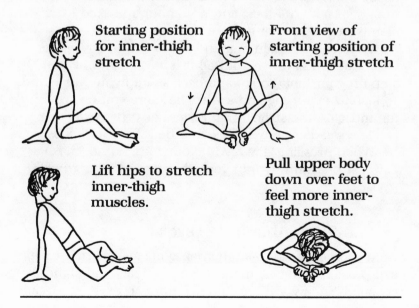

Starting position for inner-thigh stretch

Front view of starting position of inner-thigh stretch

Lift hips to stretch inner-thigh muscles.

Pull upper body down over feet to feel more inner-thigh stretch.

7 | **Your Feet**

Most people walk over their feet, not on them or with them. You should actively use your toes when walking or standing. Your toes are as useful as your fingers and should be as dextrous. And they can be, with practice.

A common and painful injury that relates to how you use your feet is called shin splints; they are caused by excess toe flexion. That means too much sudden lifting of the foot with toes up and ankle flexed, too little pressing down with the toes, and not enough relaxed extension (straightening out) of the ankle.

To lessen the pain of shin splints and to strengthen your toes, press down with all five toes each time you step on your foot. Your toe muscles wrap your ankle and so stabilize your leg and knee. The more you use your toe muscles, the stronger and steadier your ankles will be. The steadier your ankles are, the safer your knees will be. When pressing down with your toes, do not make a fist, just press firmly into your shoe or onto the ground.

Toe-Strengthening Exercise

Here is an exercise to strengthen your toes so that you can press down with them when you walk and stand. It is called "Inchworm" and comes from an exercise system developed by Bess Mensendiek, a European physical therapist. Patience and persistence are required to master this exercise, but it is well worth the trouble. It can be done sitting or standing and is best done barefoot. You use one foot at a time. First you press down the tips of all five toes, arching the area just behind them so that you lift the ball of your foot from the floor. This moves your heel forward. (When you become skillful your foot may move forward as much as an inch or two each time.) Then keep your heel in its new position and reach your toes forward so that your whole foot is flat on the floor again.

Repeat the lift of the ball of your foot and the slide of your heel forward, and reach with the toes to bring your foot flat on the ground. Keep doing this until your foot is 4–6 inches ahead of the starting point. Then with your whole foot raised slightly off the floor except for the toe tips, and keeping the arched position, pull your foot slowly back to the starting point, pressing firmly on all five toe tips. Imagine you are making long parallel toe lines in wet sand or clay. Repeat this exercise 3 times on each foot. Remember to do this slowly and don't make a fist with your toes.

When you stand or walk, point your feet straight ahead, not in or out. Gently allow your body weight to

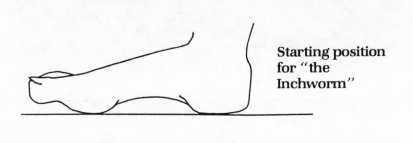

Starting position for "the Inchworm"

travel forward from your heel onto all the surfaces of your feet and especially onto all five of your toes. Pay attention to pressing down your big toe because it should be very strong. The big toe muscle is the major muscle of your main arch; the stronger this muscle is, the steadier your ankles will be. As you push forward with the foot behind you, use your toes to push yourself forward, and don't just let them bend at the joint called the ball of the foot.

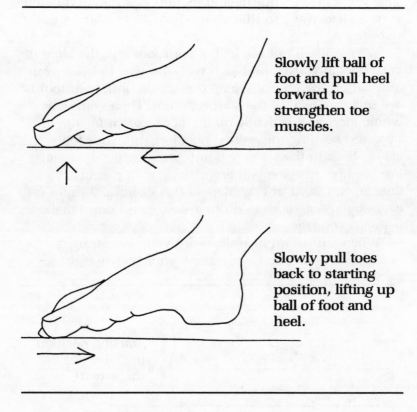

Slowly lift ball of foot and pull heel forward to strengthen toe muscles.

Slowly pull toes back to starting position, lifting up ball of foot and heel.

8 | Common Running and Walking Mistakes

Injuries occur most often as a result of continued misuse or unbalanced use of muscles. They do not just happen suddenly but build up over time. The best way to prevent injuries, therefore, is to correct bad habits, establish new ones, and maintain them.

Correct Walking

The way you walk is often the way you run. Walking and running should be like bicycling in that all three joints of your leg should work: hip, knee, and ankle.

Start your walk with your knees unlocked and your entire body weight forward over your whole foot, not just back on your heels. Feel that your body parts are stacked one on top of the other: head over shoulders, rib cage over hipbone, upper body over the whole foot, knees unlocked with legs straight. Keep your body weight forward, over the front foot, during the entire time of walking or running.

1. The first part of the walk begins with your knee leading, not your foot, and your legs swing forward and back in your hip sockets. Once you get going, your walking has three parts: the push part, the weight-transference part, and the weight-receiving part. The push part leads with your knee. This happens because you extend your

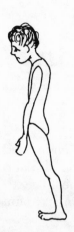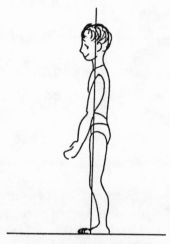

Wrong stance! for
standing, walking,
and running

Correct stance for
standing, walking,
and running

ankle and push forward with your toes as though you
were starting "Inchworm."

2. The weight-transference part occurs as you swing
your pushing foot forward. Here it is important to keep
pressing down the toes of the standing foot.

3. The weight-receiving part occurs when you set
your foot down on the ground, starting at the heel, and
put your weight straight on the entire foot with all five
toes pressing down.

Common Mistakes

Your leg should swing at the hip, forward and back. Your
bent knee (not your foot) should lead your walk, gently

bending and gently straightening. Your knee should not lock in either the weight-receiving part of your walk or run, the front part of your step, nor the push part of your step, the time when your foot is behind you. The most serious walking problem that can make your knees susceptible to injury in walking and running is swinging your leg forward with your leg entirely straight, not bent at the knee, and dropping it down on your heel. Your foot should extend at the ankle in the push part of the walk or run, with your toes pressing down and then pushing you forward. Most people who get shin splints carry each foot forward, from behind, in a flexed position. It is very im-

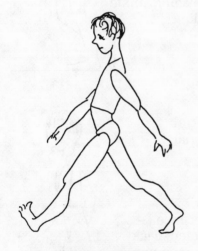

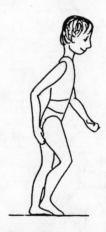

Wrong! Do not walk or run with straight legs and with body parts out of alignment.

Preparation for walking: Lead with the knee.

Partial weight
transference from
back foot to front
foot

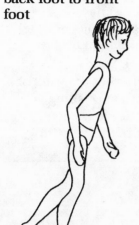

Back foot pushing
body forward,
knee leading, ankle
extending

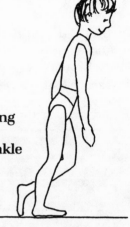

Weight-
transference part
of walk

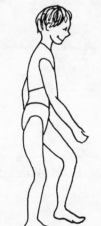

Weight
transference
completed, back
foot now comes
forward to receive
body weight.

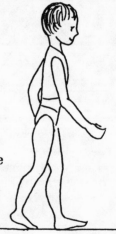

portant to extend your ankle and use your toes to press down and forward.

Walking with toes out or in prevents the knee from riding directly over the foot, where it belongs. If your knee is outside or inside your foot, and not directly over it, you will cause serious strain on the supporting ligaments and padding cartilages of your knee. You also cause uneven stress in the hip socket, and produce overtight outer thigh muscles by walking with toes out, and overtight inner thigh muscles by walking with toes in, "pigeon-toed." So, straightening out your feet when you walk can benefit your entire body.

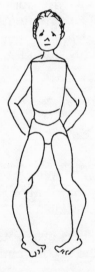

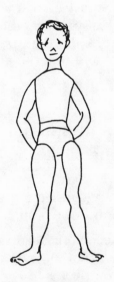

Wrong! Do not stand, walk, or run with toes in.

Wrong! Do not stand, walk, or run with toes out.

Too long a stride is another common problem that makes joints vulnerable to injury in walking and running. Shorter strides are more efficient and minimize the stress on all your leg joints and your back and neck. You can walk and run just as fast and maybe faster because in taking a short stride you can keep your body weight over your front, weight-receiving foot, where it belongs. When your upper body is still over your back foot, you have to drag it forward in an extra and straining motion in every step.

These mechanical problems should be corrected. The other major preventive measure you should take is to stretch all the leg muscles adequately before *and* after all physical exercise. First the calves, the lower part of the back of your leg; then your hamstrings, the upper part of the back of your leg, the back of your thigh; then your quadriceps, the front part of your thigh; and then your buttocks and outer thigh muscles with "the Pretzel."

Safe Running and Walking: A Checklist

When you start walking or running, it is a good idea to check very consciously where all of your body parts are in relation to each other. Here is a checklist:

1. Keep your head vertical, your ears over your shoulders, not forward and down. Bring your chin in toward your neck and look down with your eyes, not with a forward-tipped head.

2. Relax your shoulders, and feel that your shoulder blades are being pulled down with imaginary weights. When running, feel that your elbows have weights pulling them down.

3. Swing your arms front and back, not side to side, and don't twist your rib cage from side to side.

4. Feel that your whole hip moves forward and helps to initiate each step, rather than that your walk comes only from your legs.

5. Swing your thigh bone front *and* back equally at its hip joint. Many people don't allow the leg to swing back but stop the movement in a straight-down position.

6. Let your bent knee lead your walk, not your foot. Swing your leg with a bent knee and receive your weight with your knee slightly bent, not straightened and, especially, not locked. Swing your knee straight forward, not in or out.

7. Release your ankle when your foot is behind you and pushing you forward.

8. Step straight forward on your foot, not turned in or out. Keep your knee straight over your foot. Do your best to keep both feet equally straight forward (many people turn one foot out more than the other). Even a quarter of an inch turnout can place painful stress on your knee or ankle.

9. Press down your toes, especially the big toe, on each step and push yourself forward with your toes for each step. Receive your weight straight forward on your foot from the heel to all five toes; don't place your weight unevenly on the inside or the outside of your foot.

10. Take small steps and keep the upper part of your body forward over the front foot, not back over the back foot.

11. Feel pulled up from the top of your spine, which comes up into the back part of your head.

12. *Place* your feet down, don't throw them or drop them down onto the ground.

9 | In Case of Injury

There are two kinds of injuries: very severe and not so severe. For very severe ones — where you've broken a limb, severely bruised an area, or torn a muscle fiber, tendon, or ligament — you need to see a doctor immediately. He or she will treat your specific injury to enable it to heal properly. Although your doctor may not be familiar with the details of the many rehabilitative programs now available and therefore may not wish to recommend a specific rehabilitative regime, most doctors would agree that you should, if at all possible, maintain modified activity while the injury is healing in order to stay in shape.

For a not-so-severe injury — where you've mildly bruised an area or overstretched a muscle, commonly called a "pulled" muscle — you can resume gentle activity for the injured part of the body much sooner than for a severe injury.

1. Check with a doctor to make sure no bone is broken or any ligaments or tendons are torn.

2. Let it heal for 3–5 days! Do not do any activity with the injured part for 3–5 days, or until you no longer feel "Ouch!" pain in that area.

3. If possible, stretch the muscles of the area near and around the injury to prevent stiffness.

4. Resume gentle and modified activity when the pain is gone.

5. Make sure to align your body parts and stretch before and after activity.

6. Keep the injured area warm to increase blood flow to the area, because muscle, tendon, and ligament tissue soften when warm.

7. While the injury is healing, take extra time to warm it up properly *before and after* your workout.

8. After it is healed, take extra care to warm up the healed area sufficiently because, though scar tissue is stronger than normal tissue, it is also tighter. The injured area will regain its original strength and flexibility, but that process takes time.

10 | Summary

Readiness Exercises for Your Legs

6–9 minutes before *and* after

Since strenuous leg activity tightens and strengthens your legs, you need to balance this with proper stretching.

1. Calf stretch 1–2 minutes (pages 58–61).
2. Hamstring stretch 1–2 minutes (pages 62–64).
3. Quadriceps stretch 1–2 minutes (pages 68–71).
4. Pretzel stretch 1–2 minutes and underneath shoulder stretch at the same time (pages 81–83 and 40).

After leg activity, add three curl-downs to the routine, 20 seconds for each curl-down — 1 minute total (pages 52–55).

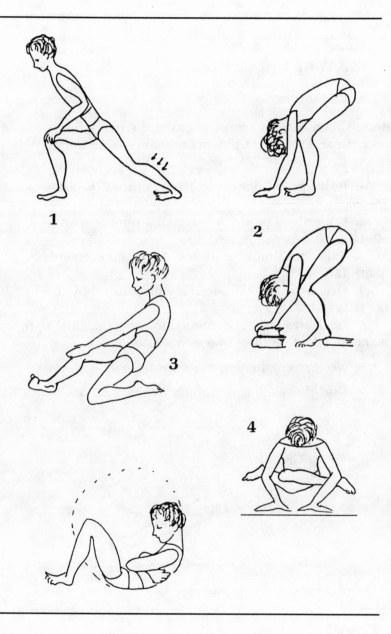

1

2

3

4

Readiness Exercises for Your Upper Body

8–10 minutes

Here is a balance of arm strength and stretch, neck strength and stretch, and a maintenance of abdominal strength.

1. Pushups — floor or wall 1–2 minutes (pages 38–39).

2. Underneath shoulder stretch 1 minute (pages 40–41).

3. Side arm shoulder stretch 1 minute each side (page 42).

4. Overarm shoulder stretch with jump rope 1 minute (pages 43–45).

5. Neck stretches — center, side, side, diagonal right, diagonal left 3 minutes (pages 30–32).

6. Neck strengthening 1½ minutes (pages 33–34).

7. Curl-downs, 3 sets 1 minute (pages 52–55).

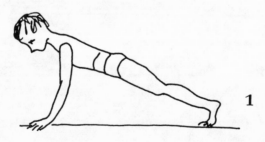

1

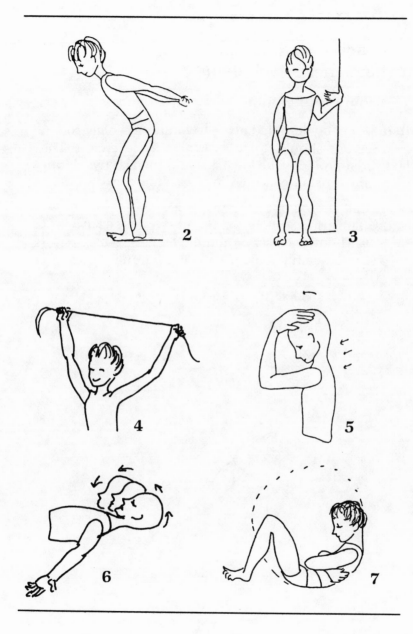

Readiness Exercises
for General Well-Being

Minimum: 7 minutes

Here is an "If-you-only-have-a-few-minutes" daily routine.

Everyone should do at least these five exercises. The first three protect your low back and the last two counteract the tension collected in your shoulders and neck.

1. Calf stretch 1–2 minutes (pages 58–61).
2. Hamstring stretch 1–2 minutes (pages 62–64).
3. Curl-downs, 3 sets 1 minute (pages 52–55).
4. Underneath shoulder stretch 1 minute (pages 40–41).
5. Center neck stretch 1 minute (page 31).

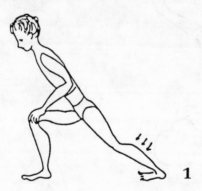

1

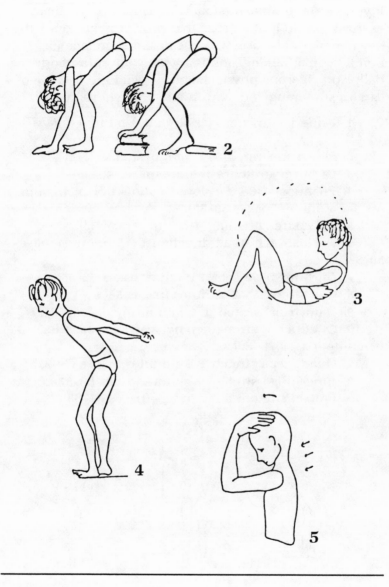

2

3

4

5

Maximum: 13–20 minutes

If you have the time, the following is a list of the best exercises to do in the order that provides your body the most comfortable, useful, and efficient sequence for building, maintaining, and readying your entire body for daily and vigorous physical activity. Note the balance of careful stretching and slow strengthening exercises.

1. Underneath shoulder stretch 1 minute (pages 40–41).
2. Side arm stretch 1–2 minutes (page 42).
3. Overarm stretch 1 minute (pages 43–45).
4. Pushups, 4–6 sets: slow 4 counts down, 4 counts up 1–2 minutes (pages 38–39).
5. Neck strengthening 1 minute (page 33).
6. Neck stretch in all directions 1–2 minutes (pages 30–32).
7. Curl-downs, 3 sets 1 minute (pages 52–55).
8. Calf stretch 1–2 minutes (pages 58–61).
9. Hamstring stretch 1–2 minutes (pages 62–64).
10. Quadriceps strengthening, 3 sets for each leg 1 minute (pages 77–80).
11. Quadriceps stretch 1–2 minutes (pages 68–71).
12. Inner-thigh stretch 1 minute (pages 86–87).
13. Pretzel stretch 1–2 minutes (pages 81–83).

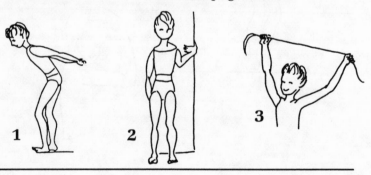

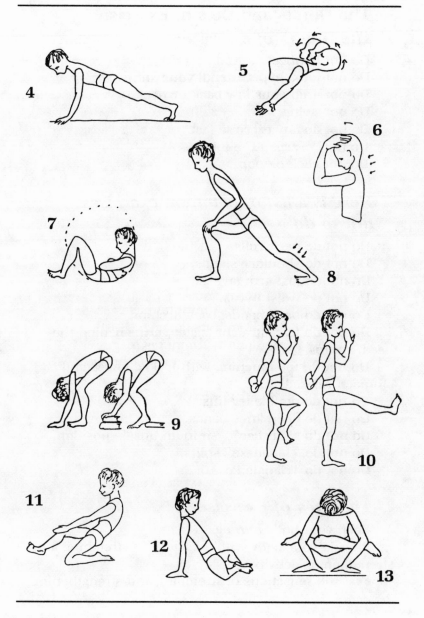

The Don'ts and Do's of Exercise

1. *The **Don'ts** of exercise:*

Do not bounce.
Do not lock (hyperextend) your joints.
Do not arch your low back or neck.
Do not swing.
Do not do any exercise fast.
Do not "overbend" a joint.
Do not click or pop.

*Here is a list of common exercises **not** to do:*

Do not do neck rolls.
Do not do shoulder stands.
Do not do fast arm swings.
Do not do waist twists.
Do not do back bends, back arching.
Do not do fast, straight-legged, arms-behind-the-head, sit-ups.
Do not do toe touching with locked knees and stomach relaxed.
Do not do double leg lifts.
Do not do deep knee bends.
Do not do "Hurdler's" sit in an unsafe position.
Do not do "Japanese" splits.
Do not do Triangle Pose.

2. *The **Do's** of Exercise*

Keep your body *moving.*
Provide your body with a *balance* of stretching and strengthening activity.
Feel the sensations of stretching and strengthening.

Stretch:

1. *Hold* the correct position for 30 seconds to a minute, or longer as necessary.

2. Actively feel the stretch in your *muscles*, not ligaments or joints.

3. Before and after any strengthening activity, stretch out the contracted muscles.

Strength:

1. Always protect your spine by putting your body parts in a safe, nonstraining position.

2. Do strengthening exercises *slowly*, moving the body part down *and* up against gravity.

3. When you are tired, do the strengthening exercise once more, carefully.

4. *Feel the exercise in your muscles*, not your joints or ligaments.

5. Guard against locking any joint.

Stop any and all exercise if it hurts, "Ouch!" hurts

Do trust your ability to distinguish between the safe feelings of stretch and strength from the harmful feeling of pain.

Do take charge of your body, its health and well-being, by keeping in motion safely. Now you know what "safely" means.

Acknowledgments

This book was written for the many people who care about their bodies, care about preventing further injury, and care about informing their families, students, teachers, and friends about how to exercise safely. I am grateful to all my students who asked questions, to the people who arranged and attended the many injury-prevention workshops that I have given, and to the people who eagerly said that I should write down the workshop material in a book.

Specifically, I want to express my deeply felt gratitude to many individuals:

— to Rochelle Robkin, who willingly drew and redrew the illustrations with such care, concern, and patience;

— to those who patiently, carefully, and wisely read the manuscript as it grew and developed: Bacia Edelman, John Olsen, Arthur A. Leath, and Ed Bersu, professor of anatomy at the University of Wisconsin Medical School;

— to John Anderson, professor of anatomy and dean of students at the University of Wisconsin Medical School, and to John Ceely, writer and friend, for the time, thought, and care that they devoted to several critical readings of the manuscript;

— to Austin Olney, editor-in-chief of Houghton Mifflin Company, for asking me to develop the initial idea of this book;

— to Dr. Rene Cailliet for his helpful comments and suggestions and Dr. Lyle Micheli for his enthusiastic endorsement;

— to Ruth Hapgood, my editor, for the energy, enthusiasm, perseverance, and intelligent care that she has shared with me in the process of working and reworking this manuscript;

— to copy editor Lois Randall for applying her wonderful ability to be precise and meticulous to the ideas and words of the manuscript;

— to designer Cope Cumpston, who skillfully and tastefully interwove the verbal and visual messages of the manuscript to form the book;

— to Debbie Ticktin, my friend, who meticulously typed several versions of the manuscript.

To *all* the people who helped me —

Thank you!

Recommended
Books for
Injury Prevention

Alter, Judy. *Stretch and Strengthen*. Boston: Houghton Mifflin Company, 1986.

Beaulieu, John E., M.A. "Developing a Stretching Program," *The Physician and Sports Medicine* 19(11):59–69 (November 1981).

Cailliet, Rene, M.D. *Low Back Pain Syndrome*. 3rd ed. Philadelphia: F. A. Davis Company, 1981.

Clarke, H. H., ed. *Physical Fitness Research Digest*. Series 6, no. 3. Washington, D.C.: President's Council on Physical Fitness and Sports, July 1976.

De Lateur, Barbara J. "Exercise for Strength and Endurance." In *Therapeutic Exercise*. 3rd ed. John V. Basmajian, ed. Baltimore: The Williams and Wilkins Company, 1978.

Drury, Blanche J. *Muscles in Action: A Kinesiological Chart of Skeletal Muscles*. Palo Alto: The National Press, 1962.

———. *Posture and Figure Control Through Physical Education*. Palo Alto: Mayfield Publishing Company, 1965.

Lagerwerff, Ellen B., and Karen A. Perlroth. *Mensendieck: Your Posture and Your Pains*. Garden City: Anchor/Doubleday, 1973.

Mensendieck, Bess M., M.D. *Look Better, Feel Better*. New York: Harper and Brothers, 1954.

Wells, Katherine F., Ph.D. *Kinesiology: The Scientific Bases of Human Motion*. 4th ed. Philadelphia: W. B. Saunders Company, 1978.

Williams, Paul C., M.D. *Low Back and Neck Pain: Causes and Conservative Treatment*. Springfield, Illinois: Charles C. Thomas, Publisher, 1974.